LAUREN HUBELE

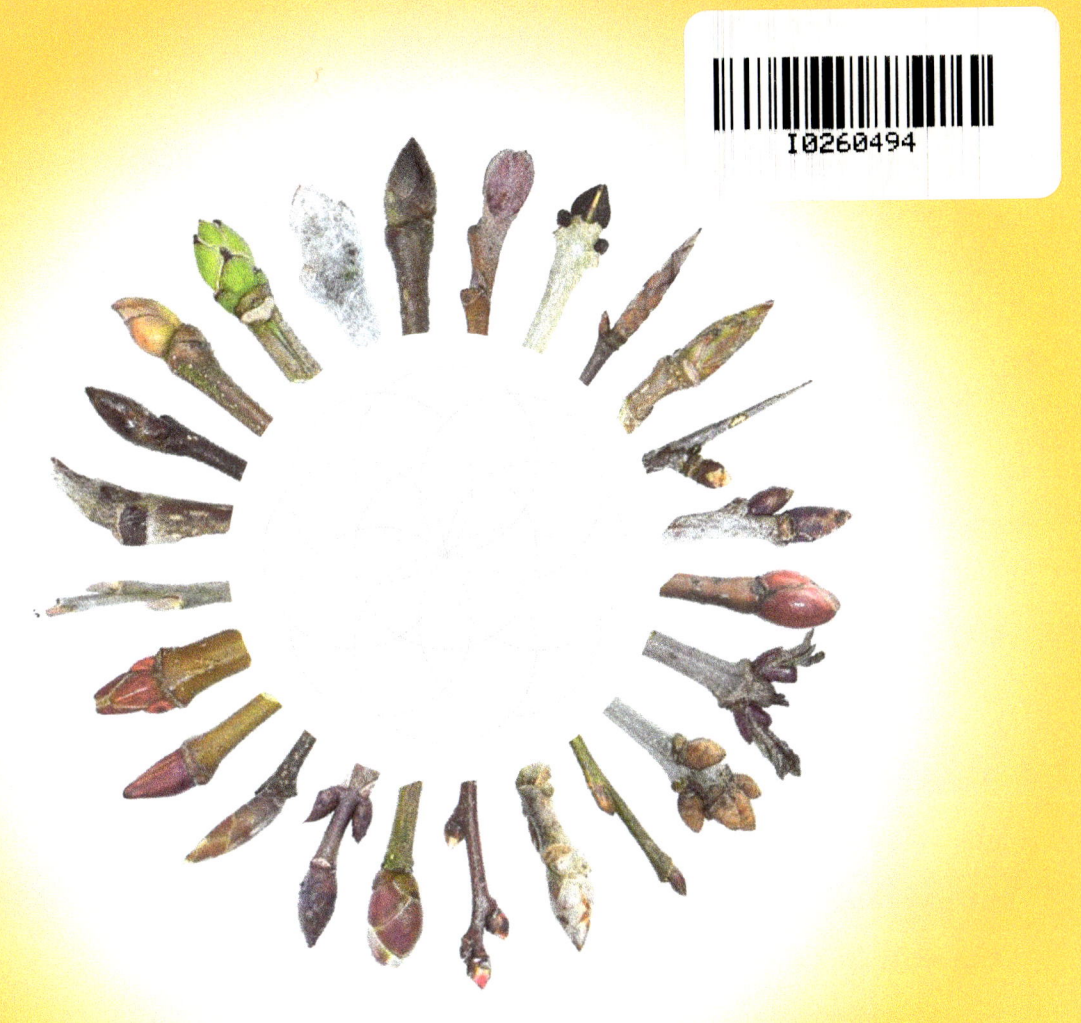

THE ART & SCIENCE OF GEMMOTHERAPY

HOW TO SUPPORT COLDS, FLU & VIRUSES

Copyright © 2025 Lauren Hubele

All rights reserved. Apart from any fair dealing for the purpose of private study, research, criticism or review, as permitted under the Copyright, Designs and Patents Act, 1988, no part of this book may be reproduced, stored or transmitted, in any form or by any means, without the prior written permission of the publishers.

ISBN 979-8-9986688-2-1

First edition 2025

Published by Gemmos with Lauren

www.laurenhubele.com
www.gemmoforest.com

About Artist Laura Roman
Laura Roman lives in Sibiu, Romania, and has been painting for as long as she can remember. It is her favorite mode of expression. She studied art and art history, and the inspiration for her creation comes from the outside world.

About Designer Christine Terrell
Art, design, and creativity coalesce into one throughline for Christine. Splitting her time between the coast of Maine and the heart of Texas, she is in constant pursuit of new ways to transform the mundane into something beautiful.

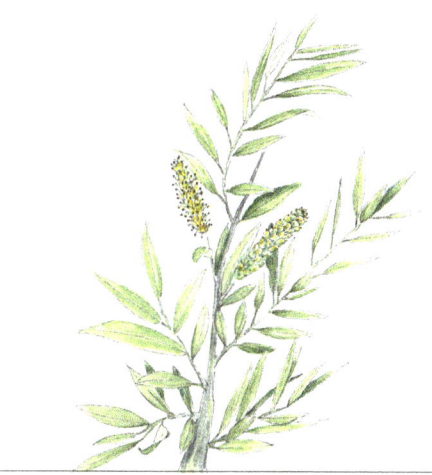

DEDICATION

This book is dedicated to the individuals and families who entrusted me with their care during my years as a health coach in Austin, Texas. Your openness and thoughtful feedback created the fertile soil which has allowed this body of knowledge to grow and mature over time. I am grateful for the opportunity and happy to be able to share the fruits of our collective efforts.

Lauren

TABLE OF CONTENTS

Getting Started — 7
Stage One: Boosting your immune response — 11
Stage Two: Supporting the body's natural cleaning process — 17
Stage Three: When secondary support is needed — 23
Stage Four: Restoring strength and vitality — 29
Extract Descriptions for Acute Care — 35

Black Currant	36	Horse Chestnut	62
Black Honeysuckle	38	Lingonberry	64
Black Poplar	40	Lithy	66
Blackthorn	42	Magnolia	68
Common Alder	44	Oak	70
Common Birch	46	Oat	72
Common Fig	48	Sea Buckthorn	74
Dog Rose	50	Silver Birch Buds	76
European Blueberry	52	Silver Birch Sap	78
Field Maple	54	Silver Lime	80
Hazel	56	Sweet Chestnut	82
Hops	58	Walnut	84
Hornbeam	60	White Willow	86

Summary of Noted Precautions for Acute Protocols — 88
Possible Aggravations — 89
Your Cold, Flu, and Virus Journal — 91

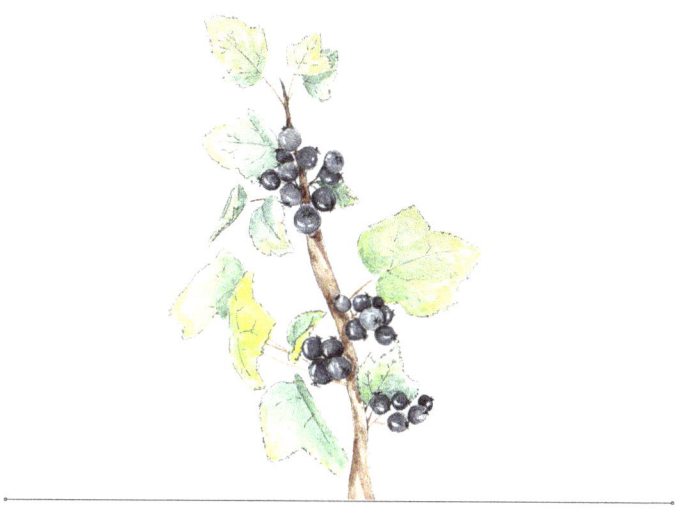

GETTING STARTED

Welcome to this wonderful world of Gemmotherapy. One of the many ways to explore the benefits of Gemmo Extracts is to use them in protocols for cold, flu, and virus symptoms. Supporting yourself and family members provides an ideal introduction to the potential these extracts hold. If you are already familiar with Gemmo Extracts, this guide can serve as a reference tool for the various stages of an acute episode and support your understanding of their remarkable synergy when combined.

It's essential, before moving further into this topic, that I take a moment to clarify the definitions of an acute symptom and an acute episode. Symptoms of acute colds, flus, and viruses come on rather quickly and are usually fast-moving. They may or may not be accompanied by a fever. They may be intense enough that you must take to your bed, but at the very least, they will slow you down for a few days.

It is also helpful to understand what are not acute symptoms. Recognizing this difference is crucial because once a symptom becomes chronic, a different approach is necessary. A cough that has lingered for weeks or months, long after a flu, is no longer acute but chronic. Continuing with a look at respiratory symptoms, seasonal allergy symptoms of the eyes and nose are chronic, as are recurring menstrual pain, migraines, or cyclical headaches. It's not uncommon for a symptom that was originally acute, such as shortness of breath, to become chronic. Determining whether it's acute or has become a chronic symptom will help determine your course of action.

This guide is specifically designed for acute symptoms. The extracts discussed are intentionally deep-acting and provide rapid responses, precisely what the body needs when addressing pathogens. These extracts, however, should never be continued once the acute episode is resolved. They may find a place in the later stages of your Gemmo journey, but for now, they should be reserved for short-term use. As the body shifts out of the intense immune response required during a cold, flu, or virus, a different type of daily support becomes necessary. Information and guidance on addressing chronic symptoms can be learned through The Gemmo School or by working directly with a trained Gemmo consultant.

Returning to the theme of acute episodes, I'd like to introduce the four stages of a cold, flu, or virus, which will be expanded upon in the preceding chapters. Each stage has its own set of Gemmo Extracts to choose from, offering the precise support needed. Familiarizing yourself with the subtle changes between each unique stage will improve your ability to create reliable and effective Gemmo protocols.

Here is a summary of the four stages:

The first stage of an acute episode is often overlooked. It is short-lived, lasting 12-48 hours, and is recognized by a subtle shift in your normal mood, energy, and appetite. The extracts for this first stage are rapid responders that are taken frequently to support that early immune response.

The second stage of an acute episode is the stage with which you will be most familiar. This is the stage at which physical expressions of acute inflammation show themselves. You will notice phlegm or mucus, drainage from the eyes, ears, or nose, a sore throat, or even the start of a cough. Alternatively, the expression could be a fever, a skin rash, loose stools, or vomiting. This stage can last anywhere from 2 to 7 days.

If your vitality is strong, inflammation levels are low, and elimination is sufficient, you may be able to bypass this **third stage** altogether. However, if those conditions are not true at the time you encounter the pathogen, then even deeper-acting extracts will be required. Secondary inflammation is the key sign that one has progressed into the third stage of an acute cold, flu, or virus, and it will continue until the vital force and elimination have improved.

The fourth stage is one of restoring resilience. This is a period of varied length during which there is a clear indication that mood, energy, and appetite have improved. During this period, the body is supported in clearing all remaining inflammation, which increases one's resilience and builds immunity against future encounters with pathogens.

Tonic and Harmonizer are two terms that you will discover in my extract descriptions. These terms relate to the quality of the message delivered by the extract to particular organs or organ systems. Understanding these terms provides another lens through which you can view the Gemmos as you develop your relationships. Note that most extracts deliver both qualities. Another way of viewing the qualities is as the Yin (harmonizing) and Yang (tonifying) messages that initiate actions.

A **harmonizing** message promotes an action similar to a friend who arrives when we are in need, rather than pushing; it simply asks, 'What is needed right now? Do you need to get out and take a walk? Or do you need to just sit here?' It'll support what you need in this moment. These harmonizing actions in Gemmos use plant intelligence to moderate their action. Because of this, these extracts can be taken for longer periods than most tonics and play a very special role in bringing the body into a state of balance.

Tonifying messages from an extract behave like a friend who says, 'Come on, it's time you're up and moving. Why don't we try going out for a run today?' The tone of the message might also be compared to that of a personal trainer.

As you can see, both friends and messages are helpful, but a tonic message when your body needs a harmonizing one can be jarring and cause aggravation. Fortunately for you, we have many years of experience supporting acute colds, flus, and viruses, so the extracts are already categorized with an appropriate timing in mind.

Now, let the following chapters lead you through the four stages of acute support. As you read, consider the last time you struggled with such symptoms and see if your memory will allow you to break the experience into similar stages.

One final disclaimer: if you are coming to this book having already experienced another framework of learning Gemmotherapy, you will note right away that the dosages I recommend appear low. Over the last decade, I've come to believe that most bodies and most circumstances require less, rather than more, Gemmo Extracts. Only in a case of secondary bacterial infections have higher doses proven more effective, but even then, that has not always been the case. As with most things in life, you won't know unless you try, and this might be an opportune time to expand your view of how Gemmos work in the body.

You will also note that I intentionally share very general guidelines for dosing, as each person and situation is unique.

As a general rule, I recommend the following:

1. Always begin with a low dose and watch for any signs of aggravation before increasing it.

2. Limit the number of extracts given within one day to no more than five for children and only up to seven for adults. Gemmos are information for the body; finding the balance of how much information is provided and how often is precisely the Art of Gemmotherapy.

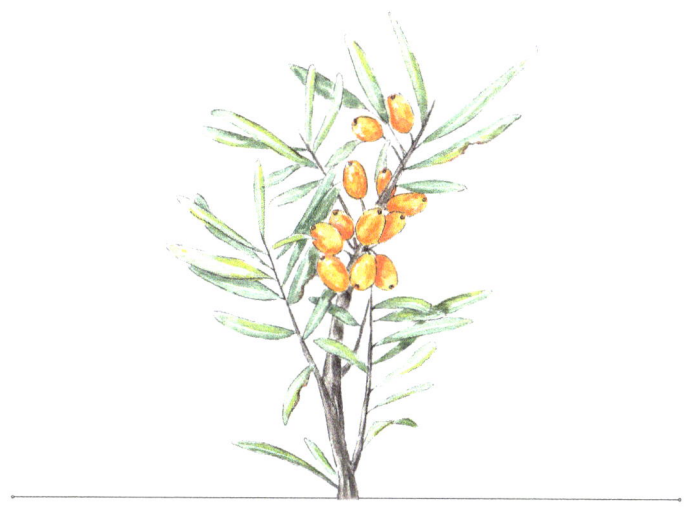

STAGE ONE
LOWERED MOOD, ENERGY & APPETITE

AT A GLANCE				
TYPICAL SYMPTOMS	EXTRACTS TO CONSIDER	DURATION	DOSING	ADDITIONAL SUPPORT TO CONSIDER
Lowered mood, energy, and appetite	Sea Buckthorn, Black Poplar, Black Currant -------- Field Maple, Oak	12- 48 hours	Take low doses (3-6 drops per extract) every 1-3 hours, reducing to 3x daily as symptoms improve or moving on to Stage Two when other symptoms appear.	Rest, increased fluids, light, easy-to-digest plant-based meals

Boosting Your Immune Response

What are the first signals you may be coming down with a cold, flu, or virus? This is the question I'll set out to answer in this chapter, as well as share the essential first extracts to take for support.

When others around you have been getting sick, you begin to feel achy or wake with a sore throat; these are all good indicators that it's a good time to take it easy and support your immune system. There are, however, other early warning signs that are more reliable. These signs appear as soon as your immune system begins its early response to a pathogen. You will experience these symptoms as a **lowered mood, decreased energy, and reduced appetite**. If the immune response is supported at this critical, early stage, the intensity and duration of symptoms will be remarkably reduced. I like to visualize the first encounter between a pathogen and your immune system as a conversation. Because the conversation and the initial response of the immune system require energy, we will experience these subtle changes in our usual mood, energy, and appetite.

Far too often, when our lives become busy and we are distracted by what feels more pressing, we miss the subtle yet essential signals our bodies communicate. Whether you become the biggest Gemmo fan or never dive into this healing modality, take away the value of noticing your mood, energy, and appetite, just like the early warning lights on your car's dashboard. These seemingly minor clues will never lead you astray and serve as no-fail indicators of the trajectory of your healing process.

It may take you a time or two to experience a cold, flu, or virus, but if you practice, your ear will become attuned to these important clues. Many adults, especially those in Western cultures, were conditioned early on not to listen to their bodies. It may be a good time now to reflect on the early conditioning you received regarding health and illness. Could some of those beliefs be ready for an upgrade?

If you are fortunate enough to have a young child in your life who has not yet been conditioned to ignore or suppress their feelings, allow them to be your teacher. An out-of-character meltdown or impromptu nap on the sofa is often a parent's first clue that something is amiss. If there was any doubt, that same child might then turn down their favorite meal or even a special treat or fall asleep at the dinner table. A wise, intuitive parent knows to expect physical symptoms to follow.

That same parent, however, may not be quite as tuned into their own needs and miss their unexpected irritability with their colleague or a desperate need to head to bed early.

I'm often asked how quickly Gemmo Extracts will work, and my answer is that it depends on the individual. How well your body responds to Gemmo support depends significantly on the level of chronic inflammation. That is why a young child experiences a much quicker response to Gemmos than a middle-aged adult who struggles with one or more chronic inflammatory symptoms.

Let's dive into the incredible support you'll find in a few very specific Gemmo Extracts for this first stage of a cold, flu, or virus. These extracts are so valuable that I dare say if you were to invest in only a handful of Gemmos, these would make the list.

Stage One Gemmos

When there is a downturn in mood, energy, and appetite, the first and primary Gemmo Extracts to consider taking in a full dose together include:

Sea Buckthorn, as an immune system tonic, offers rapid support to the immune response. It has the unique capability of altering the pH, making the site of inflammation inhospitable for pathogens to thrive.

Black Poplar is a fluid harmonizer and immune system tonic that offers a unique propolis effect, inhibiting pathogens, clearing free radicals, and resolving acute inflammatory states.

Black Currant is an Autonomic Nervous System tonic that stimulates the adrenals and the production of adrenaline and dopamine. It resolves acute inflammation with a similar effect to cortisol. It has the unique ability to amplify and improve the effect of partnering extracts.

Secondary Support as needed:

Consider adding **Field Maple** in a full dose in the late afternoon or early evening if you have a history of secondary infections. It has been proven to protect against the spread of inflammation. It is also useful if you are waking up or experiencing restless sleep between 11 pm and 3 am.

Consider adding **Oak** in the afternoon when exhaustion is a primary symptom. As an adrenal support effecting cortisol levels. It can be used in combination with **Black Currant**.

Suggested Dosing Options

Begin once first signs of:

- lowered mood
- decreased energy
- reduced appetite

Every 3 hours:

Take together in a small amount of water, **Sea Buckthorn**, **Black Poplar**, **Black Currant**. (Add **Oak** in the afternoon dose if exhaustion is severe.)

Before Sleep: **Field Maple**

OR

Every Hour:

Take individually directly on your tongue or in a small amount of water: **Sea Buckthorn**, **Black Poplar**, **Black Currant**. (Add **Oak** in the afternoon doses if exhaustion is severe.)

Before Sleep: **Field Maple**

What's Next?

One of the two things will occur within 48 hours—other symptoms will appear, or your mood, energy, and appetite is restored. If other symptoms appear, proceed to Stage 2. If restored, discontinue use of Acute extracts.

STAGE ONE OBSERVATIONS AND NOTES

STAGE ONE OBSERVATIONS AND NOTES

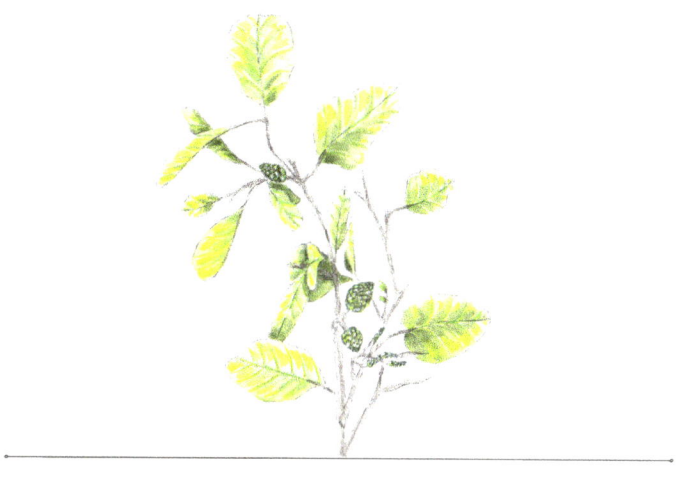

STAGE TWO
SYMPTOMS APPEAR

AT A GLANCE

TYPICAL SYMPTOMS	EXTRACTS TO CONSIDER	DURATION	DOSING	ADDITIONAL SUPPORT TO CONSIDER
Phlegm or mucus, drainage from the eyes, ears, or nose, a sore throat, or even the start of a cough, a fever, skin rash, loose stools, or vomiting.	Common Alder, Black Currant -------- Dog Rose, Hornbeam, Black Honeysuckle, Lithy, Black Poplar, Blueberry, Common Fig, Silver Birch Sap -------- Hazel, Field Maple	2-7 days	Micodose (1-2 drops) CNS extract All other extracts 3-12 drops, dependent on age and response. -------------------- Use the lowest dose to get the desired result. (Of Acute extracts, 3-18 drops -------------------- Limit the number of extracts daily to 5 for children, 7 for adults	Rest, increased fluids, light, easy-to-digest plant-based meals, or abstain from solid foods if vomiting or loose stools.

Stage Two of an acute episode is the stage with which you will be most familiar. This is the stage at which physical expressions of acute inflammation show themselves. You will notice phlegm or mucus, drainage from the eyes, ears, or nose, a sore throat, or even the start of a cough. Alternatively, the expression could be a fever, a skin rash, loose stools, or vomiting. This stage can last anywhere from 2 to 7 days.

Create a protocol that supports your current symptoms. As your symptoms progress or change, adjust your protocol accordingly, always maintaining the fewest extracts possible to address the areas that need support. (Dosing guidelines are listed with each extract description)

Common Alder and **Black Currant** are the duo you need most in stage two of all acute illnesses. **Common Alder** acts as a fluid harmonizer, balancing mucus levels and flow during this stage when mucus production is heightened. The harmonizing action is key here, maintaining moisture where it is needed and absorbing moisture where it is abundant. Its ability to improve the movement of lymph and circulation is welcome at a time when bodily fluids become congested. **Common Alder** can be used throughout the second and third stages; however, it must always be included in a complete protocol, never taken alone. If symptoms linger beyond two weeks, an extract to support elimination must be added to any protocol with **Common Alder**.

Pairing **Common Alder** with **Black Currant** boosts its effectiveness and supports the resolution of inflammatory states. Black Currant's tonic action on the Autonomic Nervous System also improves the various immune response functions.

Based on the location and intensity of the inflammation, choose from the following additional extracts for your protocol. Please read the description of each extract for further details.

SYMPTOMS	Nose & Eyes	Ears	Throat	Cough	Wheezing, Restriction of Breath, Croup	Vomiting or Frequent Loose Stools	Skin Rash
EXTRACTS TO CONSIDER	Dog Rose	Dog Rose & Blueberry	Black Honeysuckle	Hornbeam	Lithy	Fig	Silver Birch Sap

Central Nervous System Support

By supporting the Central Nervous System with an extract that acts as a harmonizer, you will improve your ability to pause and respond to your symptoms and experiences rather than react. Just one morning microdose of a Central Nervous System harmonizer will improve how this all-important sensory manager communicates with the organ systems involved in the immune response.

Select the one that best matches your current emotional state during this second stage of your illness. If your emotional state changes, adjust the extract accordingly. Take one drop directly on the tongue upon waking, separate from your other extracts.

Important note: An extract can be taken only in a microdose or full dose within a day, not both. For instance, if you are using **Dog Rose** or **Black Poplar** in full doses to address your physical symptoms, consider using one of the other four extracts in a microdose.

Dog Rose - Which supports the shift from a fragile to a supported state

Walnut - Which supports the shift from a threatened state to an engaged state

Oat - Which supports the shift from an ungrounded to a stabilized state

Hops - Which supports the shift from a state of avoidance to a fully present state

White Willow - Which supports the shift from a harried state to one of ease

Black Poplar - Which supports the shift from a state of fear to one of courage

Silver Lime - Which supports the shift from separation to connection.

Evening Support

Sleep can be challenged due to symptoms and your system being out of balance. Using the 12 hours of the evening to support immunity and your sleep can be achieved with one of the following extracts. These extracts can be microdosed if used for a sleep support only or taken in a higher dose if the immune support is needed.

Consider **Hazel** for children and adults who struggle with surrendering to a restful sleep and regularly struggle with chronic bronchitis, asthma, or pneumonia, particularly when inspiration and expiration are challenged.

Consider **Field Maple** for children over three years and adults whose mood plummets in the evening, experience night waking between 11pm and 3 am, or can benefit from extra immunity support to prevent secondary inflammation.

There are several ways you can take these extracts and find them effective. Below are two suggestions that have worked well for me and my former clients, producing good results in resolving symptoms. I suggest selecting one format as a starting place and adjusting as you learn to read your body's signs and build your relationship with the extracts.

Suggested Dosing Options:

Upon Rising: The Central Nervous System Extract **With Breakfast:** Common Alder, Black Currant, and a third extract* **Midday:** Common Alder, Black Currant, and a third extract* **Late Afternoon:** Common Alder, Black Currant, and a third extract* **After Evening Meal:** Either Hazel, Field Maple, or Hornbeam *Choose an extract that matches the central area of inflammation from the list above*	**OR**	**Upon Rising:** The Central Nervous System Extract **With Breakfast:** Common Alder, Black Currant, and Dog Rose **Mid Morning:** Black Honeysuckle, Lithy, or Hornbeam **Midday:** Common Alder, Black Currant, and Dog Rose **Late Afternoon:** Black Honeysuckle, Lithy, or Hornbeam **After Evening Meal:** Either Hazel, Field Maple, or Hornbeam As symptoms improve reduce frequency of dosage to 3x daily.

What's Next?

Most cold, flu, and virus symptoms end their cycle in this stage. If mood, energy, and appetite have returned to normal levels, then your immune system has done its job. There may be lingering mucus that will take a few days to absorb, but you are indeed ready to move on to **Stage Four** and consider a protocol to strengthen your resilience. However, if mood, energy, and appetite have not returned to normal levels and symptoms persist or worsen, additional support is certainly warranted. Refer to the **Stage Three** chapter for details on options.

STAGE TWO OBSERVATIONS AND NOTES

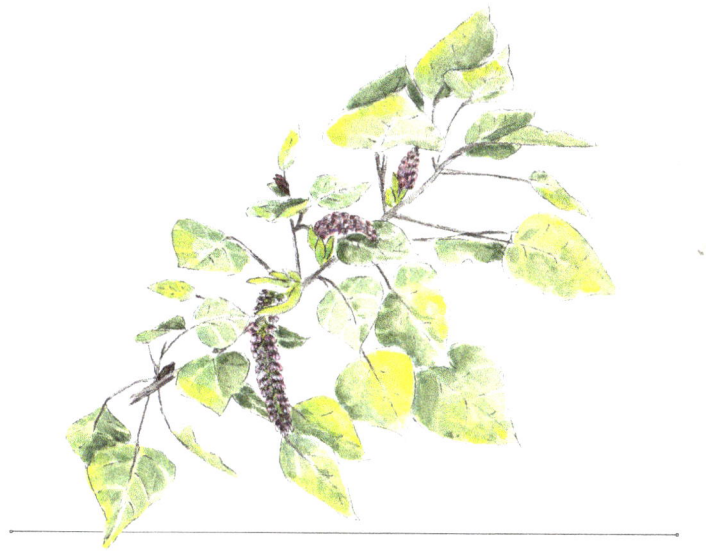

STAGE THREE
INCREASED INFLAMMATION

AT A GLANCE

TYPICAL SYMPTOMS	EXTRACTS TO CONSIDER	DURATION	DOSING	ADDITIONAL SUPPORT TO CONSIDER
Deep cough Tightness, heaviness in the chest Lethargy, fatigue, loss of hope in improvement.	Sweet Chestnut Black Poplar Horse Chestnut ---------- Field Maple Hazel	2-7 days	Micodose (1-2 drops) CNS extract All other extracts 3-12 drops, dependent on age and response. -------------------- Use the lowest dose to get the desired result. (Of Acute extracts, 3-18 drops -------------------- Limit the number of extracts daily to 5 for children, 7 for adults	Complete bed rest, increased fluids, light, easy-to-digest plant-based meals, or abstaining from solid foods if vomiting or loose stools.

Sometimes, the cold, flu, or virus pathogen cannot be neutralized and eliminated, and the inflammatory state increases and spreads rather than resolving. Stage Three of an acute illness requires the utmost care and attention. You are at your weakest state, which impairs your ability to make sound decisions and tend to your needs. If you have been on your own, tending to your symptoms, this is the time for additional support, another set of eyes to monitor your state. If you have not already consulted with your practitioner, do so. If you can access therapies that increase the vital force or Qi, include them in your self-care.

Stage Three is the time for homeopathic remedies, acupuncture sessions, or cranial sacral support, if not already included. Conventional medications may also be needed if improvement in mood, energy, or appetite does not occur. To complement the therapies mentioned, consider adding one or two of the three extracts that have the specific action of moving fluids. Each one brings something unique to your condition.

As you add extracts to your current daily protocol, you must remove some of the extracts taken in Stage Two, **keeping the maximum number of daily extracts to no more than 7**. Remember that Gemmo Extracts are information for your body, and too much information at once is overwhelming, diminishing the healing potential.

Black Poplar has two harmonizing actions that work to resolve Stage Three symptoms. As a harmonizer for the arteries, it improves the movement of oxygenated blood, particularly in the lower torso, which includes the lungs. As a moisture harmonizer, **Black Poplar** balances all fluid levels throughout the body, absorbing without drying membranes. These harmonizing actions also extend to the kidneys, increasing the elimination of uric acid.

Sweet Chestnut tones the lymphatic system, mainly in the lower torso, beginning with the lungs, and has a tonifying action on the immune system. It is a general drainer of toxins from the body, better than any extract known at this time. It combines well with other extracts that resolve inflammation, particularly **Horse Chestnut**, when a deeper action is required.

Horse Chestnut is a tonic for the vascular system, improving the function of the veins and vein walls. It effectively resolves vascular inflammation, thinning blood to prevent clotting. This tonifying action occurs in the lungs, lower torso, abdomen, and legs. It provides a deep and quick action for those who struggle with a relentless cough or fluid in the lungs.

At the same time, stool elimination is crucial to the healing process. Optimally, there will be two bowel movements daily, allowing the body to remove waste products and neutralize pathogens effectively. If your stool elimination has slowed, add one of the following extracts.

Blackthorn is indeed the extract with the broadest range of support, benefiting all ages from birth and all vitality levels. It is a tonic for the immune system, stimulating the action of immune cells, and a harmonizer for the intestines, balancing fluids and improving stool motility. Blackthorn's secondary effects include a mild tonifying and diuretic action on the kidneys, optimizing urine elimination.

Common Birch is an elimination support for adults of all vitality levels. It has a special affinity for the mature population, particularly those experiencing sluggish metabolism, low immunity, and reduced energy levels. I have found Common Birch to be an excellent, gentle general reboot for the body when symptoms of flu and viruses extend and during recovery. As a tonic for the kidneys and liver, Common Birch promotes the general drainage of waste products from the body.

Lingonberry is an elimination support for all vitality levels over the age of three years. It harmonizes the urinary tract and intestines, promoting a healthy flora balance. Recent research has proven its remarkable effectiveness in preventing *E. coli*, *Pseudomonas aeruginosa*, *Proteus mirabilis,* and *Klebsiella* pneumoniae from thriving. Lingonberry is also a tonic for the immune system, and it has a specific action on the reticuloendothelial system. It has strong antioxidant capabilities and a unique action on the degradation of the structural protein in tissue due to aging or disease, leading to the regeneration of cells and the establishment of healthy tissue.

Evening Support

Continue supporting your sleep and immunity with either **Field Maple** or **Hazel**. These extracts can be microdosed if used for a sleep support only, or taken in a higher dose if the immune support is needed.

Consider **Hazel** for children and adults who struggle with surrendering to a restful sleep and regularly struggle with chronic bronchitis, asthma, or pneumonia, particularly when inspiration and expiration are challenged.

Consider **Field Maple** for children over three years and adults whose mood plummets in the evening, experience night waking between 11pm and 3 am, or can benefit from extra immunity support to prevent secondary inflammation.

Suggested Dosing Options

Below are two samples suggesting how you might organize your Gemmo protocol during Stage Three.

Without an elimination extract

7 am: Morning microdose of a CNS harmonizer upon rising

9 am: Common Alder, Black Currant, and an extract that supports localized inflammation

11 am: Sweet Chestnut and Horse Chestnut OR Black Poplar

1 pm: Common Alder, Black Currant, and an extract that supports localized inflammation

3 pm: Sweet Chestnut and Horse Chestnut OR Black Poplar

5 pm: Field Maple or Hazel

With an elimination extract

7 am: Morning microdose of a CNS harmonizer upon rising

9 am: Common Alder, Black Currant, and an extract that supports localized inflammation

11 am: Sweet Chestnut and Horse Chestnut OR Black Poplar

1 pm: Common Alder, Black Currant, and an extract that supports localized inflammation

3 pm: Sweet Chestnut and Horse Chestnut OR Black Poplar

5 pm: Field Maple or Hazel

What's Next?

Most cold, flu, and virus symptoms end their cycle in this stage. If mood, energy, and appetite have returned to normal levels, then your immune system has done its job. There may be lingering mucus that will take a few days to absorb, but you are indeed ready to move on to **Stage Four** and consider a protocol to strengthen your resilience. However, if mood, energy, and appetite have not returned to normal levels and symptoms persist or worsen, additional support is certainly warranted. Refer to the **Stage Three** chapter for details on options.

STAGE THREE OBSERVATIONS AND NOTES

STAGE THREE NOTES

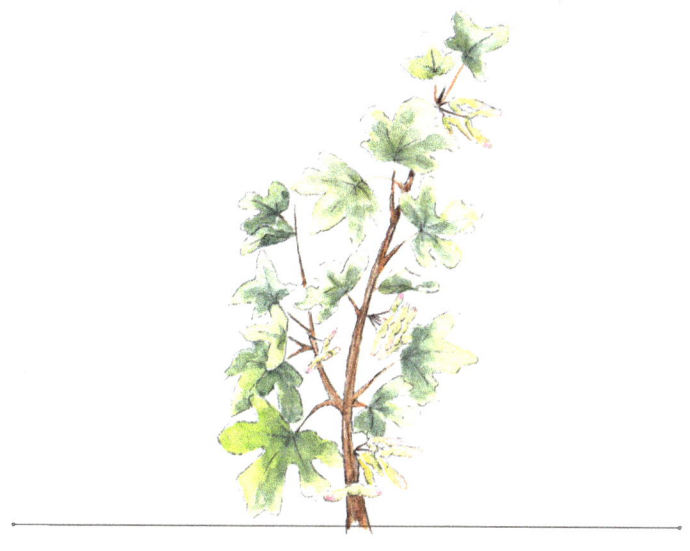

STAGE FOUR
RESTORING RESILIENCE

AT A GLANCE

TYPICAL SYMPTOMS	EXTRACTS TO CONSIDER	DURATION	DOSING	ADDITIONAL SUPPORT TO CONSIDER
Lacking usual curiosity and creativity Irritability from pushing self beyond current physical and mental limitations Fear of relapse Sluggish elimination or loose stools Loss of energy by midday, late afternoon	**For NS Support:** Black Poplar, Dog Rose, Hops, Oat, Walnut, or White Willow **For Elimination:** Blackthorn, Common Birch, or Silver Birch Buds **For Adrenals:** Black Currant or Oak **For Immune Support:** Dog Rose or Blackthorn **For Evening Support:** Field Maple or Hazel	7-21 days watching for a complete return of normal ranges of energy, appetite, and mood to signal the completion of this stage.	Acute extracts: 3-18 drops --- Nervous System extracts: 1 drop	Continue the increased amounts of fluids and support the digestive system with a diet high in fresh plant based foods.

The Fourth Stage is one of restoring resilience. This is a period of varied length (7-21 days) that continues until there is a clear indication that your mood, energy, and appetite have returned to normal levels. Your body will benefit from the continued support to clear all remaining inflammation. Gifting yourself with this additional care will increase your resilience and build immunity against future encounters with pathogens.

As with the other stages, you will be choosing extracts to match your current state, not the state you were in or the one you hope to experience.

Select extracts that:

Support your Central Nervous System

Choose one of the following six extracts that best suits your state at this moment in time:

Dog Rose - supports the shift from a fragile to a supported state

Walnut - supports the shift from a threatened state to an engaged state

Oat - supports the shift from an ungrounded to a stabilized state
Hops - supports the shift from a state of avoidance to a fully present state
White Willow - supports the shift from a harried state to one of ease
Black Poplar - supports the shift from a state of fear to one of courage

Support your Elimination

It is common for stool elimination to change during and after a cold, flu, or virus. Observe your daily pattern and choose from either **Blackthorn**, **Common Birch**, or **Silver Birch** for this period of recovery.

Blackthorn is indeed the extract with the broadest range of support, benefiting all ages from birth and all vitality levels. It is a tonic for the immune system, stimulating the action of immune cells, and a harmonizer for the intestines, balancing fluids and improving stool motility. Blackthorn's secondary effects include a mild tonifying and diuretic action on the kidneys, optimizing urine elimination.

Common Birch is an elimination support for adults of all vitality levels. It has a special affinity for the mature population, particularly those experiencing sluggish metabolism, low immunity, and reduced energy levels. I have found Common Birch to be an excellent and gentle general reboot for the body when symptoms of flu and viruses extend and during recovery. As a tonic for the kidneys and liver, Common Birch promotes the general drainage of waste products from the body.

Silver Birch Buds is an excellent elimination support for children and adults through mid-life. Its primary action is as a tonic for the immune and respiratory systems. It is effective in resolving acute and chronic inflammation in the mucosal lining of the respiratory system, promoting general detoxification of the body, and increasing metabolism. If it slows elimination, then consider one of the other extracts.

Support your Adrenals

The most common adrenal support for this fourth stage and beyond is **Black Currant**.

Oak should be considered in addition to the Black Currant if there is still considerable exhaustion.

Support your Immune Response (optional)

If you have struggled with repeated cold, flu, or virus episodes, then consider adding **Blackthorn**, **Dog Rose** or **Sea Buckthorn** for the duration of this stage.

Blackthorn offers the broadest range of support and benefits all ages from birth, and for all vitality levels. It is a tonic for the immune system, stimulating the action of immune cells. If used for elimination, it can replace an added extract for rebuilding immunity.

Dog Rose is an immune system tonic that improves the immune response and is especially useful in building immunity in children and adults with low vitality and a weakened immune system.

Sea Buckthorn is an immune system tonic that will improve the overall immune response. Its unique capability of altering the pH at the site of an inflammation offers protection against a relapse.

Evening Support

Continue supporting your sleep and immunity with either **Field Maple** or **Hazel**. These extracts can be microdosed if used for sleep support only or taken in a higher dose if immune support is needed.

Consider **Hazel** for children and adults who struggle with surrendering to a restful sleep and regularly struggle with chronic bronchitis, asthma, or pneumonia, particularly when inspiration and expiration are a challenge.

Consider **Field Maple** for children over three years and adults whose mood plummets in the evening, who experience night waking between 11 pm and 3 am, or can benefit from extra immunity support to prevent secondary inflammation.

Suggested Dosing Format

Unlike dosing during the earlier stages, the extracts you choose will only be taken once per day. Below is a sample of how a daily protocol can be organized for Stage Four:

Morning:	Midday:	After the evening meal:
A microdose of a Central Nervous System extract upon waking	An Elimination Support extract, an Adrenal support extract, and an Additional Immune extract in full doses. Blackthorn, Common Birch, or Silver Birch Buds & Black Currant (with Oak)	An extract that supports sleep and immunity, specifically Hazel or Field Maple in a microdose or full dose.

Note: If you have not seen significant improvement after 30 days, consult with your health practitioner.

What's Next?

Pause all extracts until next acute episode OR return to a daily protocol based on chronic symptoms.

STAGE FOUR OBSERVATIONS AND NOTES

_____

_____

_____

_____

_____

STAGE FOUR OBSERVATIONS AND NOTES

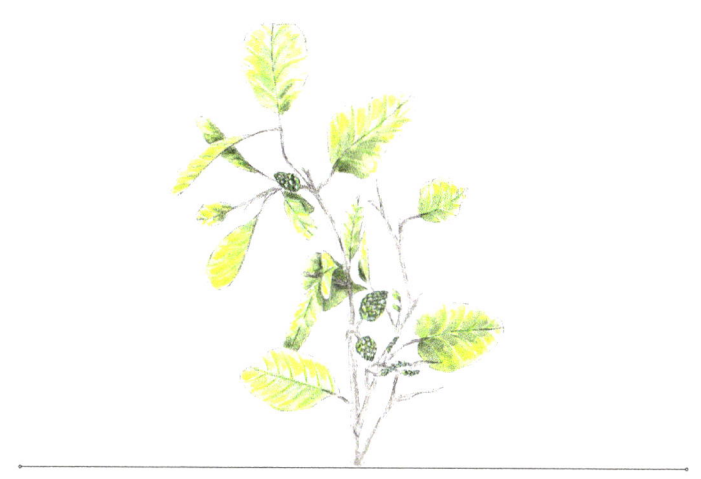

ACUTE SUPPORT EXTRACT DESCRIPTIONS

BLACK CURRANT

Ribes nigrum

The Essence: Black Currant's essence is to amplify.

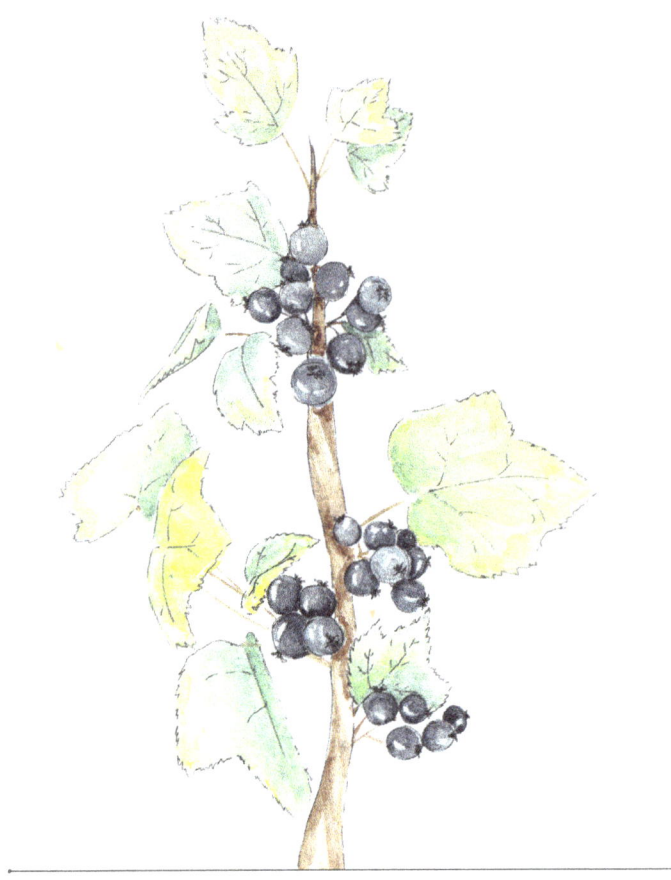

ESSENCE AMPLIFY	STAGES	1 - 4
	SUPER POWER	The ability to respond rapidly in support of the immune response and to boost the effectiveness of paired extracts is Black Currant's Super Power.
	DOSAGE	3-18 drops up to 3x daily
	AGE	From 12 months
	BEST TIME OF DAY	Anytime
	POTENTIAL PARTNERS	All extracts
	COMPARE WITH	Oak, Blackthorn
	PRECAUTIONS	No confirmed precautions at the time of publication

THE ART

Meet Black Currant

If you could own two extracts to support all acute conditions, Black Currant should certainly be your first selection because of its universal appeal, and the support it can offer all ages from birth is simply unsurpassed. The second extract would be dependent on the individual. Black Currant's rapid effectiveness and jammy taste have won over even the harshest Gemmo skeptic. It is the one extract you will use in every stage of an acute cold, flu, or virus.

As a practitioner, I found Black Currant to be irreplaceable in every mother's natural support kit. It alone got many a parent and child through a feverish night or weekend until I was available to offer a more specific protocol. Combined with Lithy, its rapid response can turn a frightening croup into a peaceful sleep for all, and with Silver Birch Sap, it can quickly resolve a viral rash or hives.

In Stage One, its tonifying effects on the Autonomic Nervous System support a rapid and effective immune response. In the second and third stages, it not only reduces inflammatory symptoms but also amplifies the effect of partnering extracts. Finally, in stage four, it increases the effectiveness of the protocol selected to restore resilience and continues to resolve any lingering inflammation.

It is most helpful for:

- Fever and body aches associated with colds, flus, or viruses on its own.
- As an amplifying extract, it is used along with additional extracts that support specific regions or organ systems.

Lauren's Experience

Black Currant is my go-to the moment I sense a reduction in my energy, appetite, or mood. I like adding it to fresh-pressed juice, herbal tea, or sparkling water when I begin to increase my fluids. I've done a fair bit of experimenting on myself over the past few years and always marvel at Black Currant's ability to amplify the effects of any extract I pair it with.

THE SCIENCE

The Actions of the Extract

Primary

The primary action of the Black Currant extract is to resolve inflammation caused by acute illness, allergies, or injuries, with an effect similar to cortisol.

Black Currant is a powerful antioxidant that clears free radicals and promotes tissue regeneration. It reduces the effects of histamines in the body, whether the response is due to food or another substance. Black Currant also stimulates the adrenals and the production of adrenaline and dopamine.

Secondary

The indirect effect of resolving inflammation produces a calming sensation.

Black Currant has been proven to amplify the actions of extracts taken along with it. Additionally the reduction of inflammation leads to an overall calming sensation.

Super Power

The ability to respond rapidly in support of the immune response and to boost the effectiveness of paired extracts is Black Currant's Super Power.

BLACK CURRANT NOTES:

_____

_____

_____

_____

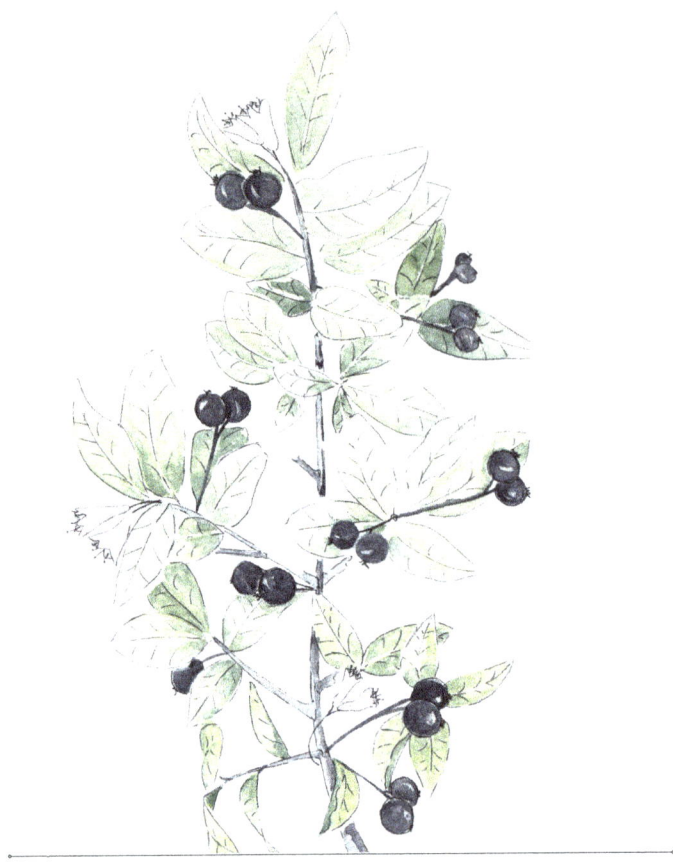

BLACK HONEYSUCKLE

Lonicera nigra

The Essence: The essence of Black Honeysuckle is fluidity.

ESSENCE FLUIDITY		
	STAGE	2 & 4
	SUPER POWER	The ability to thin phlegm and keep it moving is Black Honeysuckle's Super Power.
	DOSAGE	3-18 drops up to 3x daily
	AGE	From 3 months
	BEST TIME OF DAY	Anytime
	POTENTIAL PARTNERS	Black Currant, Common Alder, Dog Rose
	COMPARE WITH	Magnolia, Black Poplar, Hornbeam
	PRECAUTIONS	See text

THE ART

Meet Black Honeysuckle

Black Honeysuckle is a star among extracts for acute colds, flus, and viruses, and should be considered immediately in the case of an inflamed throat or post-nasal mucus drip.

Black Honeysuckle supports various acute protocols, with a particular strength in restoring health to the respiratory and intestinal mucosal membranes by thinning mucus.

- Sore throats
- Inflamed tonsils, adenoids
- Post-nasal drainage
- Thick, sticky mucus during the recovery period

Lauren's Experience

When I spent my days teaching live courses on Zoom, I would always have a bottle of Black Honeysuckle on hand to support my voice as it became fatigued. Earlier in life, pre-Gemmos, I was quite prone to laryngitis after a long day of teaching, but since using Black Honeysuckle in a preventative way, I have rarely experienced this symptom. It is, hands down, a family favorite, and was used frequently by my young granddaughter in her first years of life to soothe a sore throat.

THE SCIENCE

The Actions of the Extract

Primary

Black Honeysuckle's primary action is as a tonic for the liver and intestines, stimulating the detoxification process. It also has a direct tonifying effect on all acute inflammatory states, resolving new inflammation at the start of a viral infection and any remaining chronic post-infection inflammation. It thins mucus from the sinuses, nose, bronchi, and intestines, thereby increasing fluidity, encouraging drainage, and easing elimination.

Black Honeysuckle's ability to resolve inflammation of the throat and thin mucus offers support during acute illnesses.

Precautions

Aggravations will occur if the liver or intestines are congested and unable to clear. Observed aggravations include emotional irritability, headaches, loose stools, and hives. In those cases, an extract to harmonize the blocked organ first would be the better choice.

Super Power

The ability to thin phlegm and keep it moving is Black Honeysuckle's Super Power.

BLACK HONEYSUCKLE NOTES:

_____

_____

_____

_____

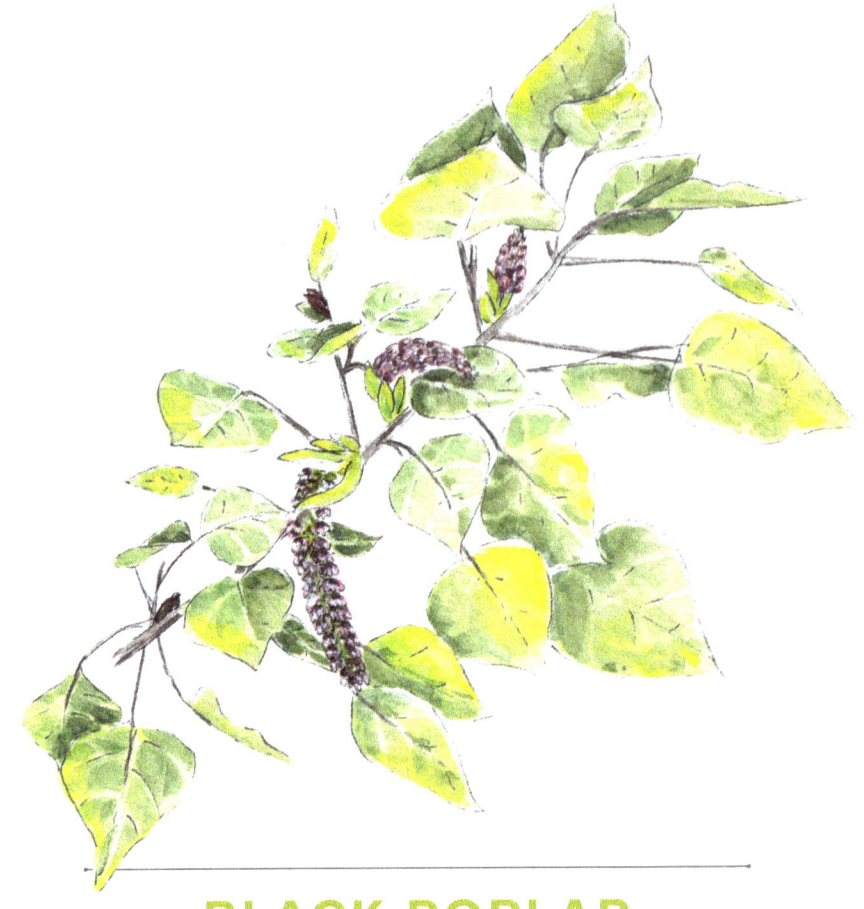

BLACK POPLAR

Populus nigra

The Essence: The essence of this essential extract is courage.

ESSENCE COURAGE	STAGE	1 - 4
	SUPER POWER	The ability to provide a unique propolis effect against pathogens is the Super Power of Black Poplar.
	DOSAGE	3-18 drops up to 3x daily
	AGE	From 6 years
	BEST TIME OF DAY	Anytime
	POTENTIAL PARTNERS	Black Currant, Dog Rose, Sea Buckthorn, Sweet Chestnut
	COMPARE WITH	Common Alder, Hazel, Sea Buckthorn
	PRECAUTIONS	See text

THE ART

Meet Black Poplar

This fluid harmonizer is best known for the prevention of inflammatory respiratory symptoms with Black Currant and Sea Buckthorn. (Mornings: Sea Buckthorn and Black Currant, Midday: Black Poplar, Late Afternoon: Sea Buckthorn and Black Currant. Then again with complementary extracts for acute respiratory inflammation when the bronchi and lungs are affected.)

I once read that Poplar is known as the tree capable of transcending fear and we have discovered the same to be true for the extract when taken in a microdose. Consider it in stages 2-4 if fear is a prominent emotion.

Lauren's Experience

As a big fan of Black Poplar, it is the one Gemmo I travel with consistently. While others may make it into my checked bag, Black Poplar is in my carry-on. I take it for its propolis effect in warding off pathogens and its harmonizing support for the kidneys, as well as its tonifying effect on the arteries, which are especially important on long-haul flights.

THE SCIENCE

The Actions of the Extract

Primary

This deep-acting extract's primary action is as a harmonizer for the arteries and as a tonic for the immune system. The arterial support is mainly in the lower body, including the lungs. Regarding immunity, Black Poplar has a remarkable propolis-like effect. The resins from the buds, similar to propolis, inhibit pathogens, clear free radicals, and resolve acute and chronic inflammatory states.

Secondary

As a moisture harmonizer, Black Poplar balances the level of fluids, helping fluids absorb without drying membranes. This harmonizing action also extends to the kidneys, increasing the elimination of uric acid. This reduction of acid improves inflammation in joints. It is a CNS harmonizer that protects the production of the neurotransmitters dopamine and acetylcholine.

Black Poplar's primary action as a tonic for the immune system, along with its propolis-like effect, helps resolve acute inflammation, while the secondary action helps balance fluids. It also acts as a harmonizer for the Central Nervous System when the emotion of fear is present.

Precautions

Due to the blood-thinning action, take only with care if using an anticoagulant medication.

Note that there are only trace levels of salicin in the extract. The highest quantity is in the bark, which is not used to make the extract. Precautions should be observed if there is a severe allergy to aspirin.

Super Power

The ability to provide a unique propolis effect against pathogens is the Super Power of Black Poplar.

BLACK POPLAR NOTES:

_____

_____

_____

_____

_____

_____

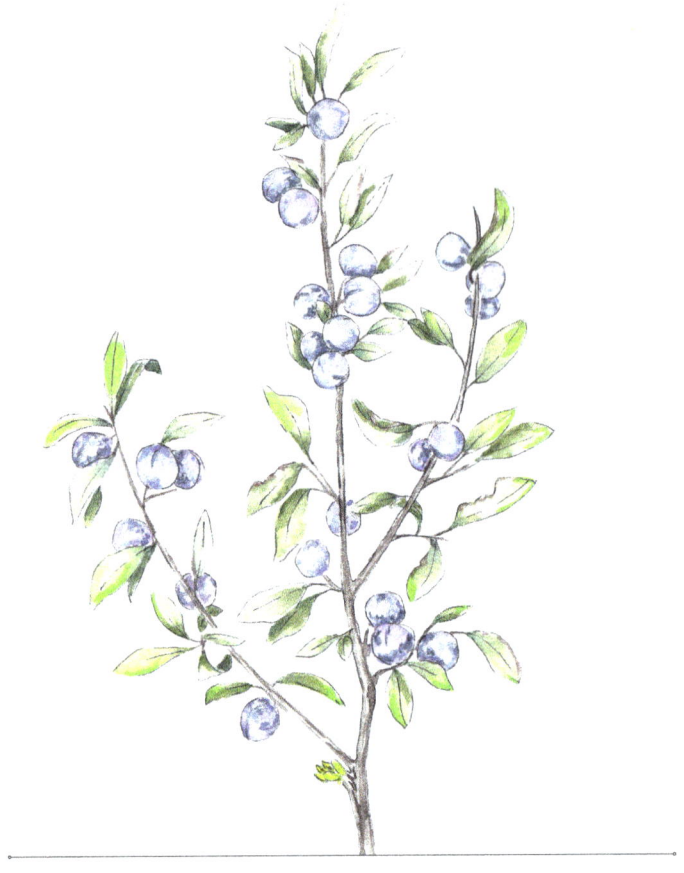

BLACKTHORN

Prunus spinosa

The Essence: Blackthorn's essence is of the protector.

ESSENCE PROTECTION	STAGE	3 & 4
	SUPER POWER	The ability to offer such widespread support to a variety of systems is Blackthorn's Super Power.
	DOSAGE	3-18 drops up to 3x daily
	AGE	From birth
	BEST TIME OF DAY	Anytime
	POTENTIAL PARTNERS	Black Currant
	COMPARE WITH	Common Birch, Oak, Silver Birch Buds
	PRECAUTIONS	See text

THE ART

Meet Blackthorn

Blackthorn is indeed the extract with the broadest range of support. Beginning with the fact that it can benefit all ages, from birth, and all levels of vitality and stool type, gives you a sense of its capabilities.

It effectively supports elimination in long-standing colds, flus, and viruses, and during stage four, it can shorten the recovery period. You must be aware, however, that when a system has not cleaned itself optimally for years or a lifetime and is suddenly reminded of how to do so, there could be a telltale sign of minor skin inflammation, indicating a lower dose or less frequent dosing is necessary. A loss in stamina during an acute illness is certainly an excellent indicator for Blackthorn.

Lauren's Experience

I turn to Blackthorn to support my elimination during an extended flu or virus. I appreciate the wide spectrum of actions and can feel its support immediately. There is also so much that Blackthorn offers the subtle body in the form of protection that I welcome as my strength returns and I begin to re-engage with the world.

THE SCIENCE

The Actions of the Extract

Primary

It provides energy to harmonize the mental and physical development of the entire body and the synthesis of hormones. It is also a tonic for the immune system, stimulating the action of immune cells.

Blackthorn's primary action is to provide energy and stimulate the action of the immune cells supports the convalescent stage of an acute cold, flu, or virus.

Precautions

If stool elimination is not occurring daily, begin in a microdose and slowly build up to a higher dose only once stool frequency improves to avoid aggravations due to the antioxidant action.

Super Power

The ability to offer such widespread support to a variety of systems is Blackthorn's Super Power.

BLACKTHORN NOTES:

_____

_____

_____

_____

_____

COMMON ALDER

Alnus glutinosa

The Essence: The essence of Alnus glutinosa is movement.

ESSENCE **MOVEMENT** 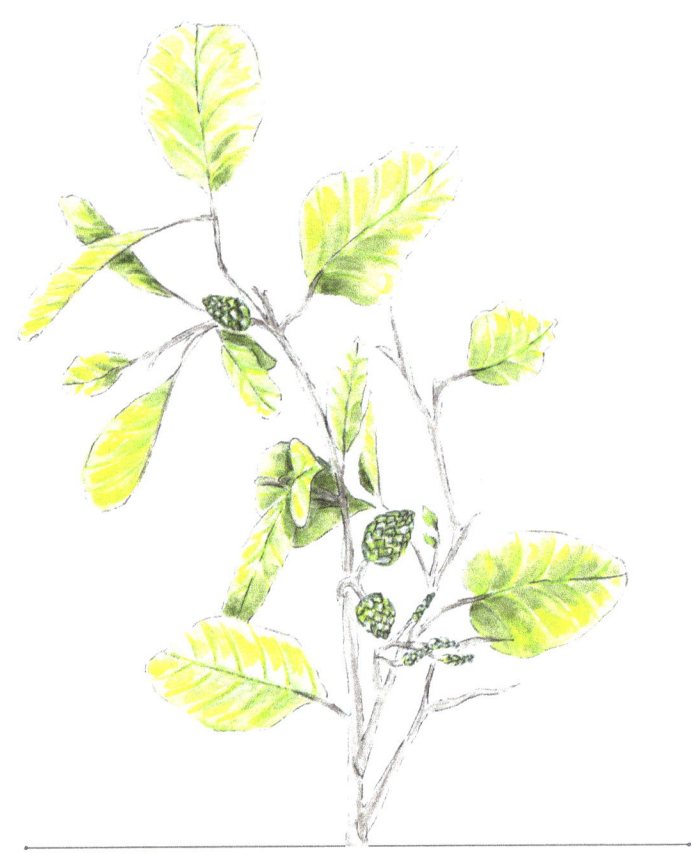	STAGE	2 - 4
	SUPER POWER	The ability to harmonize fluids right from the start of inflammation is Common Alder's Super Power.
	DOSAGE	3-18 drops up to 3x daily
	AGE	From 6 weeks
	BEST TIME OF DAY	Anytime
	POTENTIAL PARTNERS	Black Currant, Common Fig, Dog Rose, All respiratory extracts
	COMPARE WITH	Black Poplar, Sweet Chestnut
	PRECAUTIONS	See text

THE ART

Meet Common Alder

When a cold, flu, or virus has produced inflammatory phlegm, Common Alder is one of the first extracts to consider. As a team player, it should only be taken with other extracts, specifically Black Currant, to resolve the inflammatory state. Then an extract should be used to support the specific area inflamed, whether it be the sinuses or eyes (Dog Rose), throat (Black Honeysuckle), or bronchi (Hornbeam). Common Alder is a fluid harmonizer that helps the body absorb excess fluids produced during an acute state and prevents scar tissue from forming.

This beneficial extract is safe for all ages beyond six months. Keep in mind that its action is to move fluids, and when using it for longer than a week, the kidneys should be supported with an elimination extract.

Common Alder is key in all acute protocols (with Black Currant, Dog Rose, or other regionally specific extracts).

Lauren's Experience

Common Alder was one of the first Gemmos I identified as a candidate for Acute protocols because of its rapid ability to regulate fluids. I personally feel a calming effect when taking Common Alder, which could be energetic and physical. Once any mucus appears, it becomes a staple in my acute dosing of Gemmos.

THE SCIENCE

The Actions of the Extract

Primary

This extract's primary action is as a fluid harmonizer, balancing mucus levels and flow. This makes it an essential extract at the onset of inflammation. The balancing actions prevent the buildup of scar tissue by supporting fluid absorption. It also improves the movement of lymph and circulation.

Common Alder's primary action of harmonizing fluids and balancing mucus at the onset of inflammation helps support the body in absorbing excess fluids during the acute stage of a cold, flu, or virus.

Precautions

Common Alder should never be taken alone; it is meant to be combined with organ-specific extracts.

Not to be taken during pregnancy or breastfeeding, as it can reduce milk production.

Super Power

The ability to harmonize fluids right from the start of inflammation is Common Alder's Super Power.

COMMON ALDER NOTES:

_____

_____

_____

_____

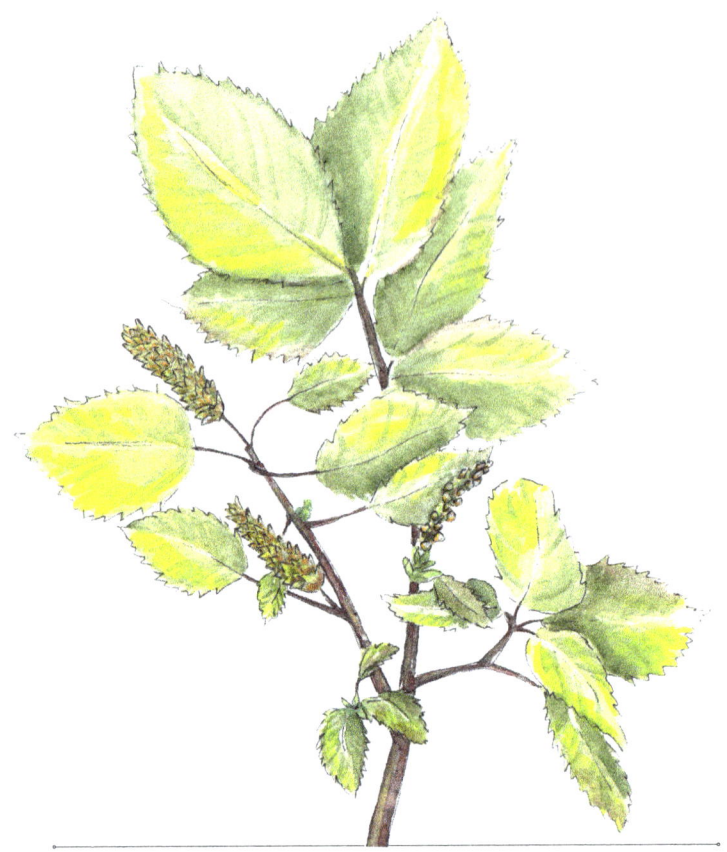

COMMON BIRCH

Betula pubescens (alba)

The Essence: The essence of Common Birch is to revitalize.

ESSENCE REVITALIZE	STAGE	3 & 4
	SUPER POWER	The ability to promote effective drainage of metabolic waste is Common Birch's Super Power.
	DOSAGE	3-18 drops up to 3x daily
	AGE	Adults
	BEST TIME OF DAY	Morning or Midday
	POTENTIAL PARTNERS	Black Currant, Lingonberry, All respiratory extracts
	COMPARE WITH	Black Poplar, Blackthorn, Silver Birch Buds
	PRECAUTIONS	No confirmed precautions at the time of publication

THE ART

Meet Common Birch

Common Birch helps support elimination for adults during an active respiratory infection and throughout the recovery period. It can also be used as an elimination support when flu and virus symptoms persist and during the recovery period. It has a special affinity for the mature population, particularly those experiencing sluggish metabolism, low immunity, and reduced energy levels. I have found Common Birch to be an excellent, gentle general reboot for the body.

Lauren's Experience

I love the restorative effects Common Birch offers my system and tend to turn to it at the end of the 4th stage of convalescence. For me, Common Birch forms a sturdy connection between what my body needs while addressing a pathogen, and what it will require on a daily basis.

THE SCIENCE

The Actions of the Extract

Primary

As a tonic for the kidneys and liver, Common Birch promotes the general drainage of waste products from the body.

Secondary

The secondary action is on the immune system, activating macrophage cells in the liver. These cells are highly effective at consuming and eliminating toxins, viral pathogens, and diseased cells. Activating macrophage cells stimulates strengthening actions in the bones, maintaining minerals, and linking calcium and phosphorus into the bones. It has general antioxidant qualities.

The secondary action of eliminating toxins, viral pathogens, and diseased cells supports adults during the recovery period of an acute cold, flu, or virus.

Super Power

The ability to promote effective drainage of metabolic waste is Common Birch's Super Power.

COMMON BIRCH NOTES:

_____

_____

_____

_____

_____

_____

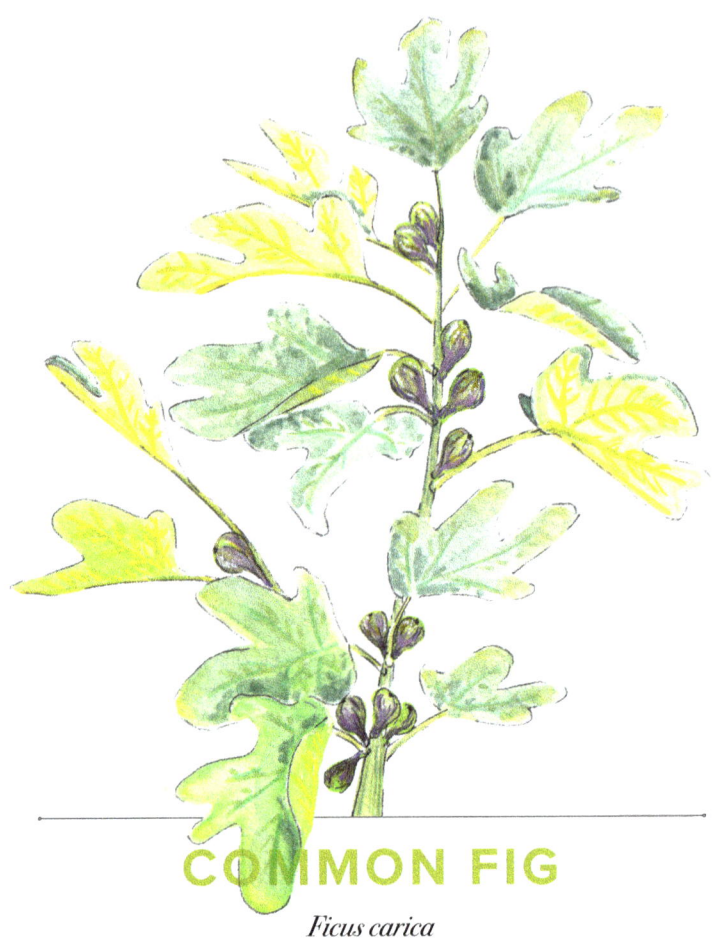

COMMON FIG
Ficus carica

The Essence: The essence of Fig extract is to process. In a microdose, Fig supports the processing of sensory input and emotions. A full dose of Fig supports the processing of food through the digestive tract.

ESSENCE TO PROCESS		
	STAGE	2 & 3
	SUPER POWER	The ability to harmonize the vagal connection to digestion is Fig's Super Power.
	DOSAGE	3-18 drops up to 3x daily
	AGE	From birth
	BEST TIME OF DAY	Anytime
	POTENTIAL PARTNERS	Common Alder, Black Currant, Walnut
	COMPARE WITH	Walnut
	PRECAUTIONS	No confirmed precautions at the time of publication

THE ART

Meet Common Fig

Common Fig is very useful in acute protocols for symptoms of nausea, vomiting, and loose, frequent stools accompanying a cold, flu, or virus. The quick action of Fig does require some monitoring, as it can halt the release of stool at a crucial time when it is necessary for eliminating pathogens and metabolic waste.

Lauren's Experience

I am not so prone to inflammatory digestive symptoms, but when they do occur, I have found Fig to be irreplaceable. It is fast-acting, and I find I only need it for a short stretch of time, but there is no other Gemmo that can match the support it offers.

THE SCIENCE

The Actions of the Extract

Primary

The primary action of Common Fig is as a Harmonizer for the Autonomic Nervous System, specifically the brain and stomach axis. There is also a noted relationship in which there is support for the transmission of acetylcholine and the function of the vagus nerve.

This harmonizing action slows acid secretion and motility of the stomach, which in turn slows digestion and stool elimination. Improvement from the Fig extract will be evident in the ability to digest food, as well as in the processing of sensory input on a mental and emotional level. A harmonizing action on the acidic pump also inhibits the histamine receptor, making this extract useful in reducing allergic reactions to foods.

Common Fig's support for loose stools, nausea, and vomiting makes it useful during acute colds, flus, and viruses.

Super Power

The ability to harmonize the vagal connection to digestion is Fig's Super Power.

COMMON FIG NOTES:

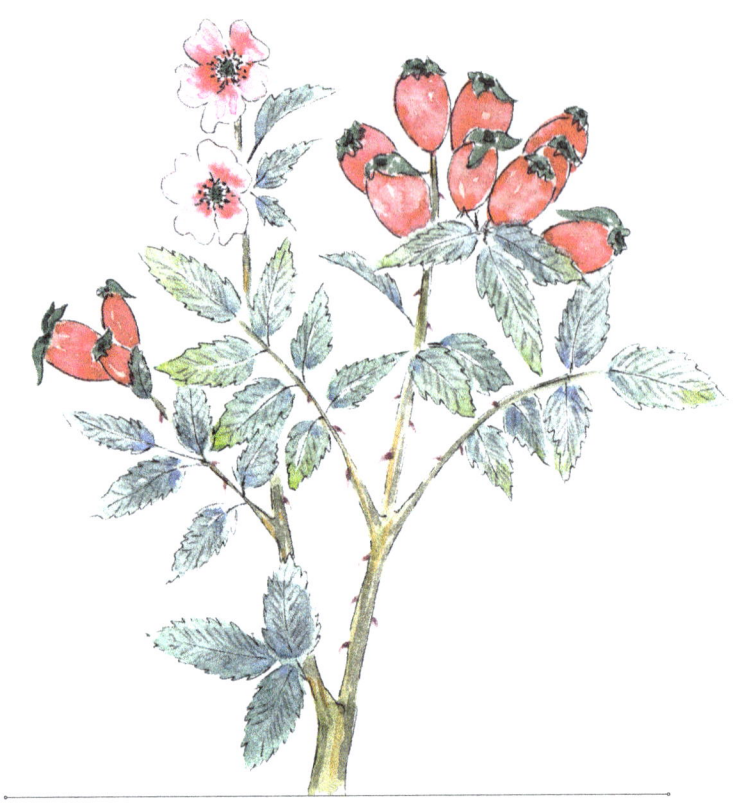

DOG ROSE

Rosa canina

The Essence: The essence of Dog Rose is its ability to effectively support even the most fragile states without causing symptom aggravation.

ESSENCE **FRAGILITY**	STAGE	2 - 4
	SUPER POWER	The ability to provide gentle support to the most fragile states is Dog Rose's Super Power.
	DOSAGE	3-18 drops up to 3x daily or 1 drop 1x daily
	AGE	From birth
	BEST TIME OF DAY	Anytime
	POTENTIAL PARTNERS	Common Alder, Black Currant, Silver Fir, Black Poplar, Sea Buckthorn
	COMPARE WITH	Sea Buckthorn
	PRECAUTIONS	No confirmed precautions at the time of publication

THE ART

Meet Dog Rose

Add Dog Rose to protocols with Common Alder and Black Currant for acute upper respiratory illnesses involving the head, adenoids, and mucosal lining of the mouth, sinus, or respiratory tract.

Use for acute headaches (with Common Alder and Black Currant—and if nausea is present, Common Fig).

Lauren's Experience

I wish I had known the benefits of Dog Rose years ago when fragile states were my norm. I can imagine it would have been a constant companion. Today, it forms a steadfast partnership with Common Alder and Black Currant in my go-to protocol for the first signs of phlegm or mucus.

THE SCIENCE

The Actions of the Extract

Primary

Dog Rose is a tonic for the immune system. It activates the immune system's first line of defense, mobilizing the macrophage cells in the respiratory and osteoarticular systems. The macrophage cells, a type of white blood cell, can engulf and destroy all pathogens in their path, making this an essential extract at the beginning stages of a cold, flu, or virus.

In addition, it resolves allergic reactions and inflammation of the mucosal lining of the mouth, respiratory, and sinus areas, as well as reducing histamines (although not as effectively as Black Currant).

Its primary action as a tonic for the immune system makes Dog Rose essential at the onset of a cold, flu, or virus.

Super Power

The ability to provide gentle support to the most fragile states is Dog Rose's Super Power.

DOG ROSE NOTES:

_____

_____

_____

_____

_____

_____

_____

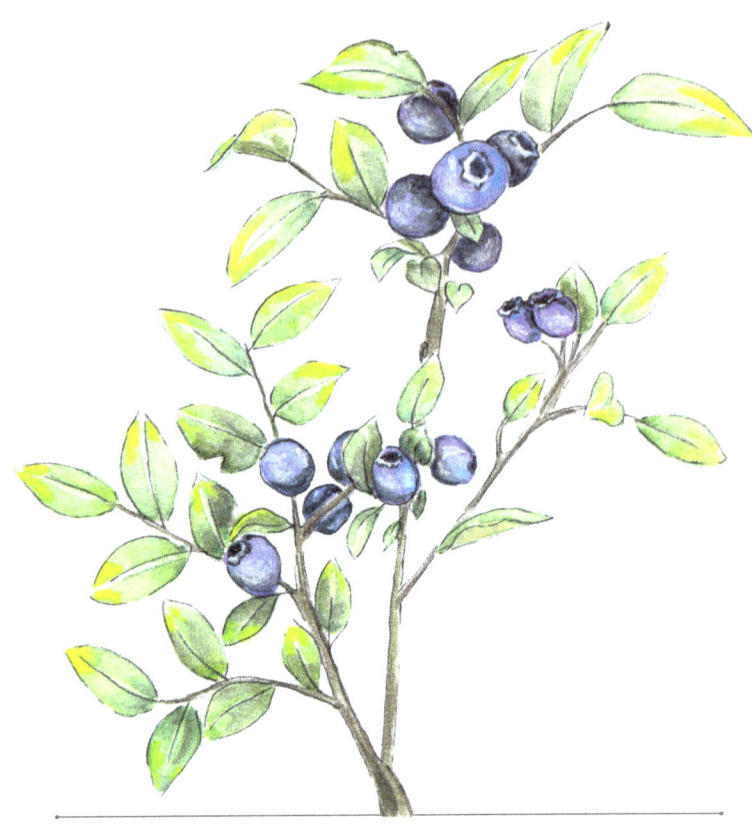

EUROPEAN BLUEBERRY

Vaccinium myrtillus

The Essence: The essence of European Blueberry, rebalance, speaks to its beautiful, harmonizing nature.

ESSENCE REBALANCE	STAGE	2 - 4
	SUPER POWER	The ability to improve microcirculation in the head is Blueberry's Super Power.
	DOSAGE	3-18 drops up to 3x daily
	AGE	From birth
	BEST TIME OF DAY	Anytime
	POTENTIAL PARTNERS	Dog Rose, Black Currant, Common Alder
	COMPARE WITH	Blackthorn
	PRECAUTIONS	No confirmed precautions at the time of publication

THE ART

Meet Blueberry

It directly supports the resolution of most acute inflammatory conditions of the ears and eyes. Indirectly, it has supported many individuals with acute flares of asthma.

European Blueberry is one member of a tried and true protocol with Common Alder and Dog Rose to resolve the symptoms of ear inflammation associated with colds, flus, or viruses. It is also to be considered as an effective support for elimination if needed in Stage 3.

Lauren's Experience

I turn to Blueberry extract for two symptoms during acute colds, flu, and viruses. My primary use is at the first sign of pressure or congestion in my ears. The secondary use is upon the first sign of my elimination slowing down. In both cases, Blueberry earns high marks and always exceeds my expectations.

THE SCIENCE

The Actions of the Extract

Primary

Blueberry is primarily a tonic for the intestines, regulating stool motility and improving flora.

Secondary

Blueberry has two secondary actions: the first is as a tonic for microcirculation in the head, strengthening vein walls in the eyes and ears, and the second is as a mild diuretic on the kidneys.

Its secondary action as a tonic for microcirculation in the head offers support to acute ear and eye inflammation.

Super Power

The ability to improve microcirculation in the head is Blueberry's Super Power.

BLUEBERRY NOTES:

___

___

___

___

___

___

___

___

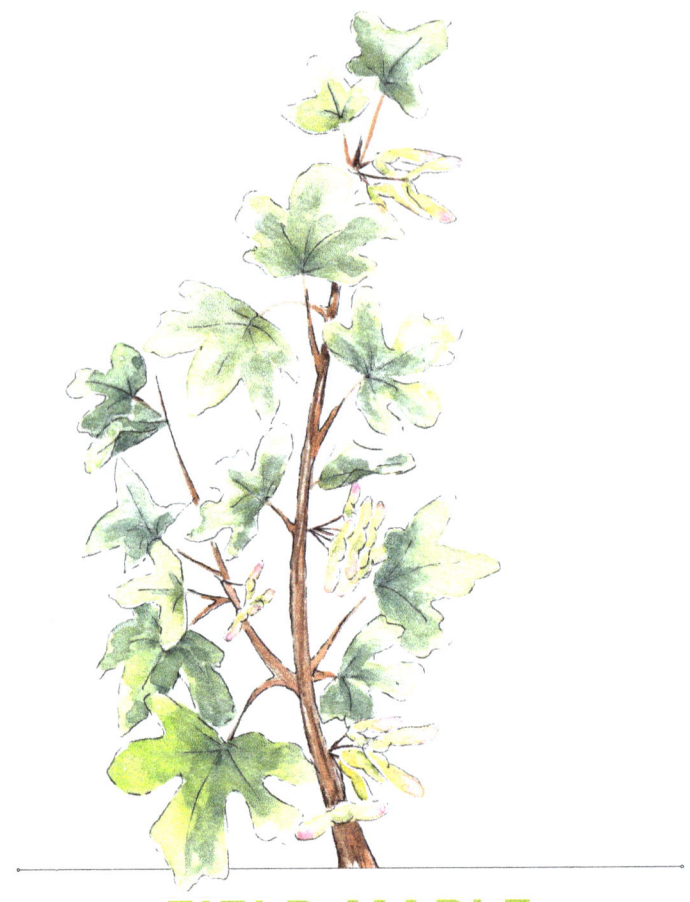

FIELD MAPLE

Acer campestre

The Essence: Access to sweetness is the essence of Acer campestre.

ESSENCE **SWEETNESS**	STAGE	1 - 4
	SUPER POWER	The ability of Field Maple to offer its unique protection against pathogens is its Super Power.
	DOSAGE	3-18 drops once daily
	AGE	From 18 months
	BEST TIME OF DAY	Afternoon, evening
	POTENTIAL PARTNERS	Common Alder, Black Currant, Dog Rose, Black Poplar
	COMPARE WITH	Hazel, Lingonberry
	PRECAUTIONS	As with all extracts for the liver, begin with a small dose and watch for aggravations such as irritability or hives.

THE ART

Meet Field Maple

With the latest research on the properties of Field Maple, it should now be considered as a primary extract at all stages of bacterial and viral infections. From the onset, to inhibit the multiplication of pathogens within the cell and throughout treatment, to protect against the spread of secondary inflammation.

Lauren's Experience

I must say that I am a huge Field Maple fan, and when it comes to the added protection it offers, it is a steady travel companion. I also find that Field Maple helps me settle into deep sleep more easily when I'm struggling with acute cold, flu, and virus symptoms.

THE SCIENCE

The Actions of the Extract

Primary

Field Maple's newly discovered tonic action on the Immune System is of great importance, offering protection against viral and bacterial pathogens.

The protection that Field Maple offers to stop the spread of secondary inflammation makes it essential at the beginning of a cold, flu, or virus.

Super Power

The ability of Field Maple to offer its unique protection against pathogens is its Super Power.

FIELD MAPLE NOTES:

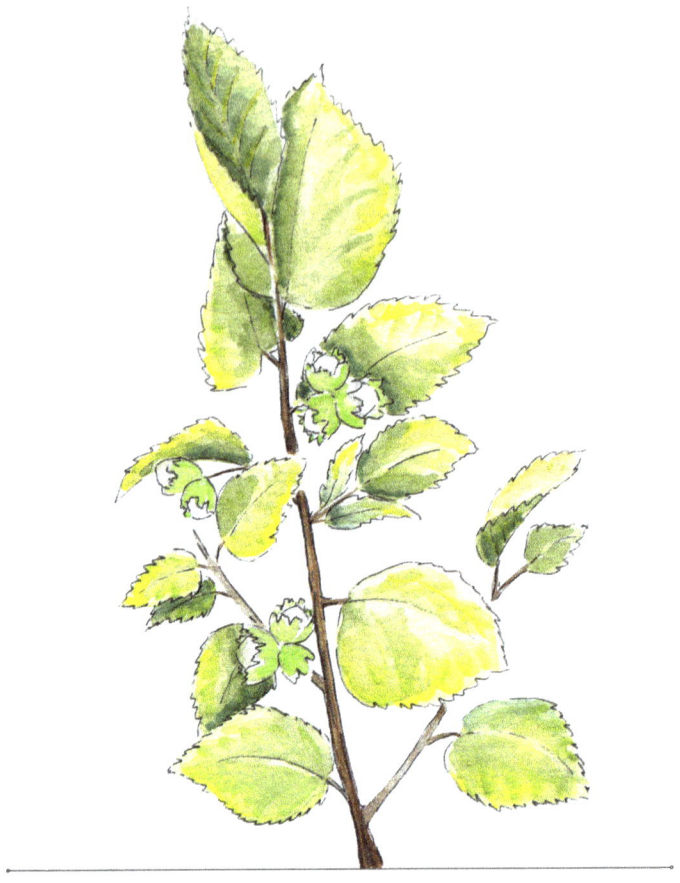

HAZEL

Corylus avellana

The Essence: The essence of Hazel extract is to soothe.

ESSENCE TO SOOTHE	STAGE	2 - 4
	SUPER POWER	The ability of Hazel to release constriction is its Super Power.
	DOSAGE	3-18 drops up to 3x daily
	AGE	From birth
	BEST TIME OF DAY	Anytime
	POTENTIAL PARTNERS	Black Honeysuckle, Common Alder, Black Currant, Horse Chestnut, Hornbeam, Lithy, Blackberry
	COMPARE WITH	Lithy
	PRECAUTIONS	No confirmed precautions at the time of publication

THE ART

Meet Hazel

Think of Hazel when the lungs are involved. Its ability to soothe and resolve inflammatory states when inspiration and expiration are challenged is unsurpassed. Hazel helps resolve acute symptoms involving the respiratory system, particularly inflammation of the bronchi and lungs. It is also an excellent extract during convalescence from colds, flus, and viruses.

Lauren's Experience

When taking a deep breath requires effort, Hazel is the Gemmo I turn to. It not only increases elasticity in the lungs but also offers soothing support to the Nervous System. I find Hazel to be a most comforting extract to take during a cold, flu, or virus.

THE SCIENCE

The Actions of the Extract

Primary

The primary action of Hazel is as a tonic on the liver and lungs, resolving inflammation of connective tissues as they lose elasticity. Results from Hazel will look like improved expiration and inspiration for the lungs and more elasticity in the liver tissue, which would be visible on scans.

Secondary

The secondary action of Hazel is as a Harmonizer for the Autonomic Nervous System and the connection with the liver, lungs, and brain.

Hazel's primary action as a tonic to resolve inflammation of the bronchi and lungs makes it an excellent choice for addressing acute colds, flus, and viruses.

Super Power

The ability of Hazel to release constriction is its Super Power.

HAZEL NOTES:

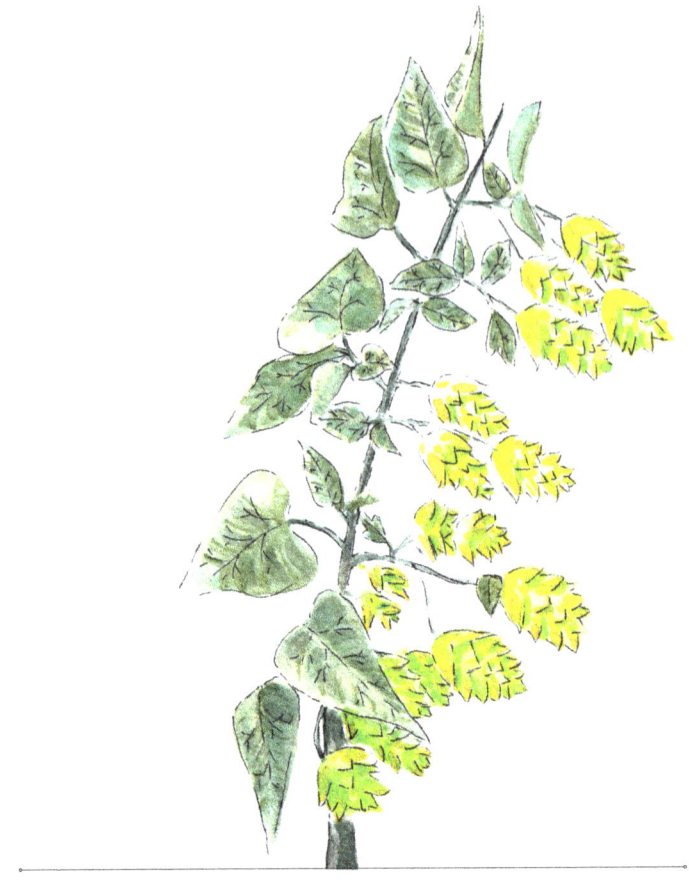

HOPS

Humulus lupulus

The Essence: The essence of Hops is to stabilize.

ESSENCE **STABILIZE**	STAGE	2 - 4
	SUPER POWER	The ability of Hops to return you to the here and now while providing a a sense of safety is its Super Power
	DOSAGE	1 drop 1x daily
	AGE	From 6 years
	BEST TIME OF DAY	Morning or Evening
	POTENTIAL PARTNERS	All acute extracts
	COMPARE WITH	White Willow
	PRECAUTIONS	See text

THE ART

Meet Hops

Think of Hops as a Central Nervous System support when a sense of disassociation is experienced during an acute cold, flu, or viral infection.

Lauren's Experience

My cue that Hops would be a welcome support during an acute cold, flu, or virus is that I catch myself scrolling my phone. It's understandable that the present isn't a comfortable place when experiencing the aches and pains of an acute illness however, awareness is critical to accurately support your symptoms.

THE SCIENCE

The Actions of the Extract

Primary

The primary action is as a sedative harmonizer of the CNS. Its specific action is on the GABA receptors, the neurotransmitters that send chemical messages through the brain and the nervous system, involved in regulating communication between brain cells.

Secondary Action

The secondary action of Hops is as a harmonizer of the ANS, supporting the ability to fall asleep. The mild harmonizing action on the endocrine system makes it useful for menopausal women.

Precautions

It's best to restrict the use of Hops to 30 days, giving it a pause for a week or more.

Hops extract does have a generalized estrogenic effect and should be avoided by all with a history of estrogen-dependent cancer.

Super Power

The ability of Hops to return you to the here and now while providing a sense of safety is its Super Power.

HOPS NOTES:

HORNBEAM

Carpinus betulus

The Essence: Taking effective action, both physically and emotionally, is the essence of the Hornbeam extract.

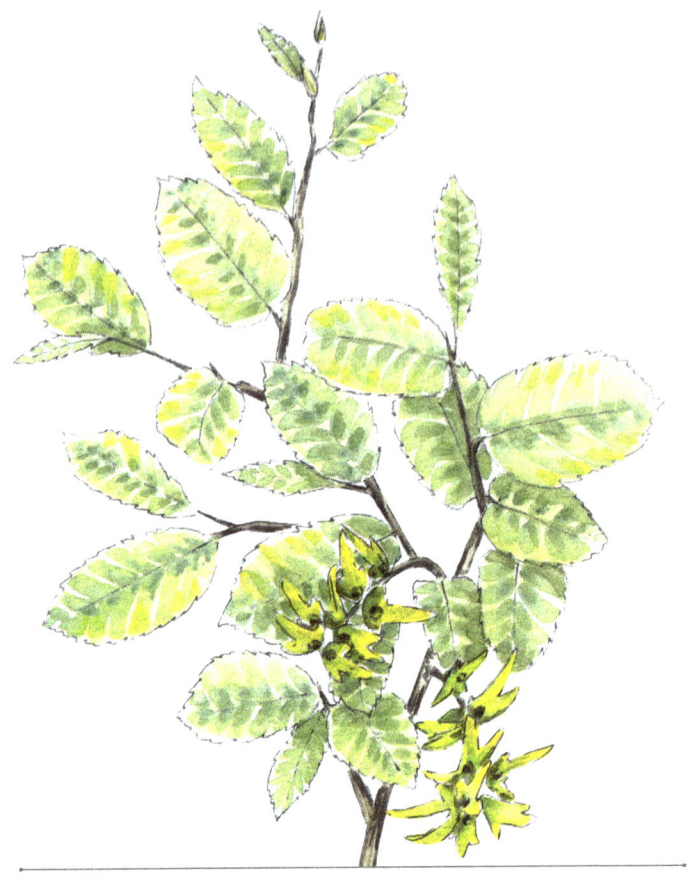

ESSENCE EFFECTIVE ACTION	STAGE	2 - 4
	SUPER POWER	The ability to harmonize a cough's effectiveness is Hornbeam's Super Power.
	DOSAGE	3-18 drops up to 3x daily, Limit to 3 weeks
	AGE	From birth for short-term use
	BEST TIME OF DAY	Anytime
	POTENTIAL PARTNERS	Common Alder, Black Currant, Black Poplar, Magnolia
	COMPARE WITH	Hazel, Lithy, Black Honeysuckle
	PRECAUTIONS	See text

THE ART

Meet Hornbeam

Use Hornbeam protocols to resolve daytime coughs associated with colds, flus, and viruses, along with Common Alder and Black Currant, or by itself or in combination with Hazel to prevent a cough that is disruptive to sleep. Due to its action on the Autonomic Nervous System, it is especially useful for irritating non-productive coughs, but can be used to improve the productivity of all coughs. In combination with Common Alder and Black Currant, it forms a synergistic action that harmonizes fluids, reduces inflammatory states, and resolves the need to cough.

Its ability to increase blood platelets cannot be overlooked, leading to my recommendation that it be used only briefly: 1 week at a time for children under three years old and no more than 3 weeks without a pause for older children and adults.

Lauren's Experience

There is no replacement for Hornbeam's ability to calm a cough that just won't stop. My favorite time to use Hornbeam during an acute cold, flu, or virus is in the evening to support a restful sleep.

THE SCIENCE

The Actions of the Extract

Primary

Hornbeam's primary action is a harmonizer for the entire Respiratory System: the sinuses, nose, throat, bronchi, and lungs. It reduces inflammation and heals existing scar tissue in the Respiratory System. Hornbeam has a unique dual action on coughs:

- It helps thin mucus, much like an expectorant.

- It will also tonify the Autonomic Nervous System, improving the effectiveness of each cough, whether mucus is too thick or resolving the need to cough when there is no mucus to clear.

Hornbeam's harmonizing action on the Respiratory System makes it beneficial during an acute cold, flu, or virus, especially when a cough develops.

Precautions

Due to its effectiveness in increasing platelet count, this extract should not be taken for more than 4-6 weeks.

There is a coagulant quality that would be contraindicated for those using anticoagulant medications.

Super Power

The ability to harmonize a cough's effectiveness is Hornbeam's Super Power.

HORNBEAM NOTES:

_____

_____

_____

_____

_____

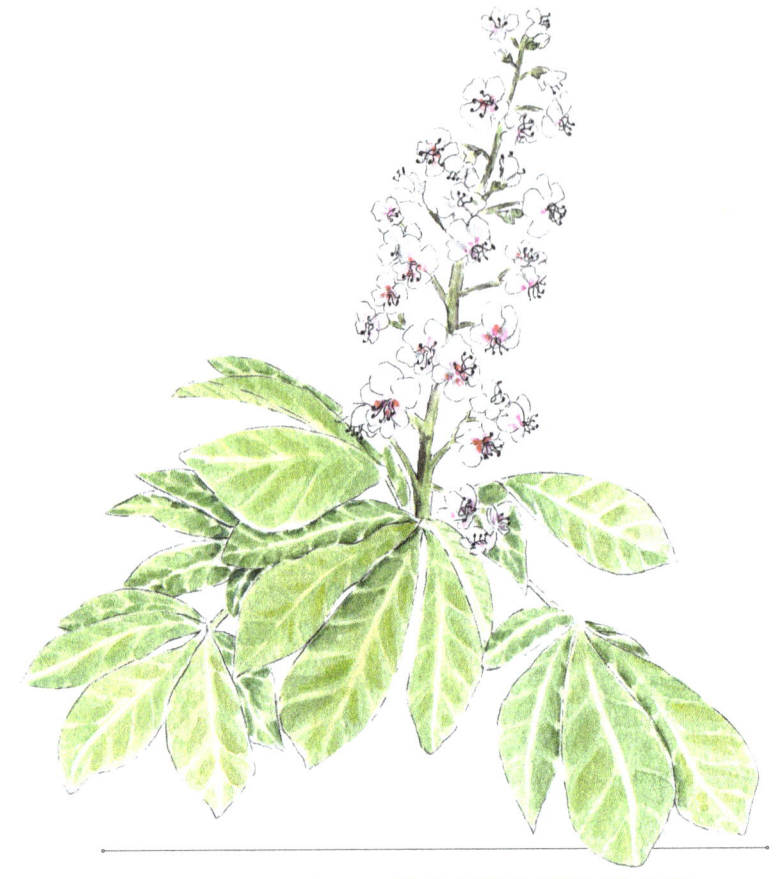

HORSE CHESTNUT

Aesculus hippocastanum

The Essence: The essence of Horse Chestnut is to decongest.

ESSENCE DECONGEST	STAGE	3
	SUPER POWER	The ability to efficiently move what is blocked is Horse Chestnut's Super Power.
	DOSAGE	3-18 drops up to 3x daily
	AGE	From 12 years
	BEST TIME OF DAY	Anytime
	POTENTIAL PARTNERS	Sweet Chestnut, Hornbeam, Common Alder, Black Currant
	COMPARE WITH	Black Poplar
	PRECAUTIONS	Not to be taken with anti-coagulant medications or daily aspirin.

THE ART

Meet Horse Chestnut

Consider Horse Chestnut to support the movement of congestion of the lungs during an acute flu or virus when other protocols are unsuccessful. Use in combination with Black Currant and other well-matched extracts such as Common Alder, Black Honeysuckle, Hornbeam, or Black Poplar.

Both Sweet Chestnut and Horse Chestnut earned their place as reliable resources during the first year or so of the coronavirus. Horse Chestnut's deep and relatively quick action provided relief for many who struggled with a relentless cough or fluid in the lungs. So, think of it when the first line of respiratory extracts fails to resolve symptoms of congestion in the bronchi and lungs.

Lauren's Experience

I've yet to need the strength of Horse Chestnut, but I've observed its effectiveness in others, and it's one powerful extract. Like Oak, a little goes a long way. Remain alert to whether the congestion has moved, and then be prepared to change to another well-suited replacement.

THE SCIENCE

The Actions of the Extract

Primary

The primary action of Horse Chestnut is as a tonic for the vascular system, improving the function of the veins and vein walls. It effectively resolves vascular inflammation, thinning the blood to prevent clotting. This tonifying action occurs in the lungs, lower torso, abdomen, and legs.

Indirect Effects

Improved circulation through the lungs and lower torso.

The tonic action for the vascular system supports the movement of congestion in the lungs during an acute flu or virus, when other protocols are unsuccessful.

Super Power

The ability to efficiently move what is blocked is Horse Chestnut's Super Power.

HORSE CHESTNUT NOTES:

_____
_____
_____
_____
_____
_____
_____

LINGONBERRY

Vaccinium vitis-idaea

The Essence: Regenerative is the essence of Lingonberry extract.

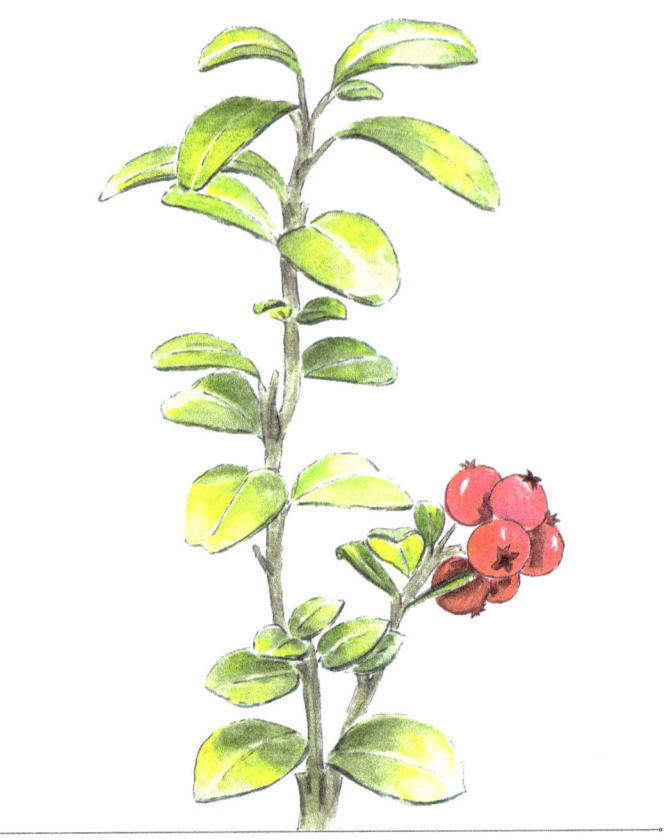

ESSENCE REGENERATIVE	STAGE	3 & 4
	SUPER POWER	The ability to rebalance and restore the urinary and intestinal systems is Lingonberry's Super Power.
	DOSAGE	3-18 drops once daily
	AGE	From 3 years
	BEST TIME OF DAY	Morning or Midday
	POTENTIAL PARTNERS	Black Currant, other acute support extracts
	COMPARE WITH	Blueberry, Blackthorn, Common Birch
	PRECAUTIONS	See text

THE ART

Meet Lingonberry

Consider Lingonberry as a primary elimination support during Stage 3 and 4 of an acute cold, flu, or virus. It is particularly important for mature individuals because of its restorative qualities.

Include in every protocol when a hospital stay is involved because Lingonberry offers protection from *Klebsiella pneumoniae*.

Lauren's Experience

When I first began working with Gemmos, Blueberry was my go-to for elimination support; however, having matured, I now find myself reaching for Lingonberry. Its harmonizing actions, particularly for older adults, make it a must-have. Since recent research revealed its tonic action on the immune system it has become part of my Gemmo travel kit.

THE SCIENCE

The Actions of the Extract

Primary

The primary actions of Lingonberry extract are plentiful. There is a harmonizing action on the urinary tract and intestines. This action promotes a healthy flora balance, and recent research has proven its remarkable effectiveness in preventing *E. coli*, *Pseudomonas aeruginosa*, *Proteus mirabilis*, and *Klebsiella pneumoniae* from thriving.

The tonic actions are on the Immune System.

The harmonizing actions on the urinary tract and intestines from Lingonberry offer support for elimination during acute colds, flus, or viruses. It should also be included in every hospital stay to protect against *Klebsiella pneumoniae*.

Precautions

It is not recommended for individuals with suspicion of or diagnosed with estrogen-dependent cancers due to its potential to increase estrogen levels.

Super Power

The ability to rebalance and restore the urinary and intestinal systems is Lingonberry's Super Power.

LINGONBERRY NOTES:

_____
_____
_____
_____
_____

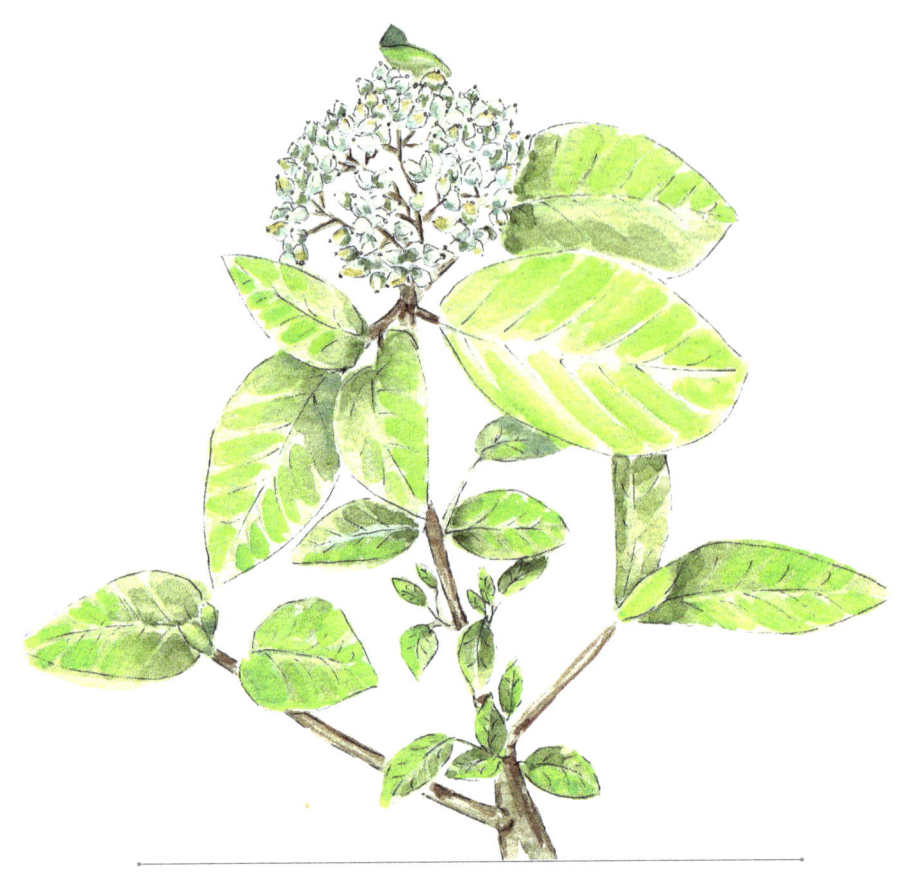

LITHY

Viburnum lantana

The Essence: The essence of Lithy extract is expansion.

ESSENCE **EXPANSION**	STAGE	2 - 4
	SUPER POWER	The ability to rapidly dilate the bronchi with a harmonizing effect is Lithy's Super Power.
	DOSAGE	3-18 drops up to 3x daily
	AGE	From 1 year
	BEST TIME OF DAY	Anytime
	POTENTIAL PARTNERS	Black Currant, Common Alder, Hazel, Hornbeam, Black Poplar, Magnolia
	COMPARE WITH	Hazel, Magnolia
	PRECAUTIONS	It can slow stool elimination, so combine it with a well-matched elimination extract when taking it daily.

THE ART

Meet Lithy

Along with other complementary extracts (such as Black Currant, Common Alder, Black Poplar, Hazel, or Hornbeam), it supports acute symptoms of the lungs and bronchi when spasms are involved.

Think of Lithy at times of restriction. This can be observed in the physical body with acute or chronic restrictive breathing in all ages and stages of life. It has remarkable qualities that can be life-changing for those who have become dependent on bronchial inhalers. This dependency extends beyond physical boundaries and significantly impacts the sense of trust and autonomy.

Lauren's Experience

Lithy is my go-to when I hear the first sign of a wheeze or a croup-like cough that causes the urge to gag. It was probably one of the most suggested extracts during my years practicing in Austin. Seasonal allergies can often cause secondary respiratory inflammation, and Lithy was a literal lifesaver for many.

THE SCIENCE

The Actions of the Extract

Primary

The primary action of Lithy is as a Harmonizer for the Respiratory System, dilating the bronchi to ease inspiration and expiration. It effectively resolves allergic reactions that cause bronchial spasms and harmonizes the contraction and relaxation of the smooth muscle cells.

The harmonizing action of Lithy on the Respiratory System allows for expansion of the lungs and bronchi when spasms are involved during acute symptoms of a cold, flu, or virus.

Super Power

The ability to rapidly dilate the bronchi with a harmonizing effect is Lithy's Super Power.

LITHY NOTES:

_____

_____

_____

_____

_____

_____

_____

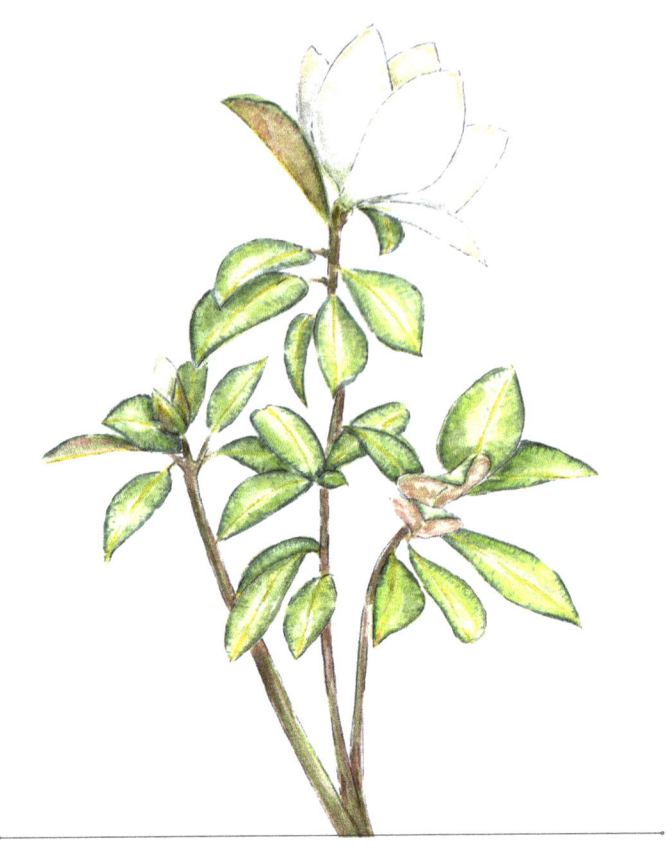

MAGNOLIA

Magnolia grandiflora

The Essence: Magnolia's essence is to resolve.

ESSENCE **TO RESOLVE**	STAGE	2 & 3
	SUPER POWER	The ability to partner with other extracts to effectively reduce inflammatory states when the digestive and respiratory systems are both involved is Magnolia's Super Power.
	DOSAGE	3-18 drops up to 3x daily
	AGE	From birth
	BEST TIME OF DAY	Anytime
	POTENTIAL PARTNERS	Black Currant and all elimination extracts
	COMPARE WITH	Common Birch, Oak
	PRECAUTIONS	See text

THE ART

Meet Magnolia

Combine with Lithy or Dog Rose, when added respiratory support is needed, or Fig if the primary concern is digestive inflammation caused by a cold, flu, or virus. A superb partnering extract, it boosts effectiveness while offering its own unique support.

Lauren's Experience

Magnolia is a new friend, and I am still getting acquainted with it when it comes to its acute support. It wasn't an extract that was available during my time as a practitioner, so my experience is limited to recent times. I have found it to be a strong and willing partner to all extracts with actions on the respiratory and digestive systems. I believe it forms a healing bridge between systems when one is needed.

THE SCIENCE

The Actions of the Extract

Primary

This extract's primary action is as a tonic for the respiratory and digestive systems, resolving inflammation of the mucosal linings, including inflammatory responses from an allergic reaction.

The tonic action of Magnolia on the respiratory and digestive systems helps resolve acute inflammation caused by a cold, flu, or virus.

Precautions

It is meant to be combined with other extracts as a partnering extract.

Avoid use during pregnancy due to the potential of trace alkaloid compounds.

Super Power

The ability to partner with other extracts to effectively reduce inflammatory states when the digestive and respiratory systems are both involved is Magnolia's Super Power.

MAGNOLIA NOTES:

_____

_____

_____

_____

_____

_____

_____

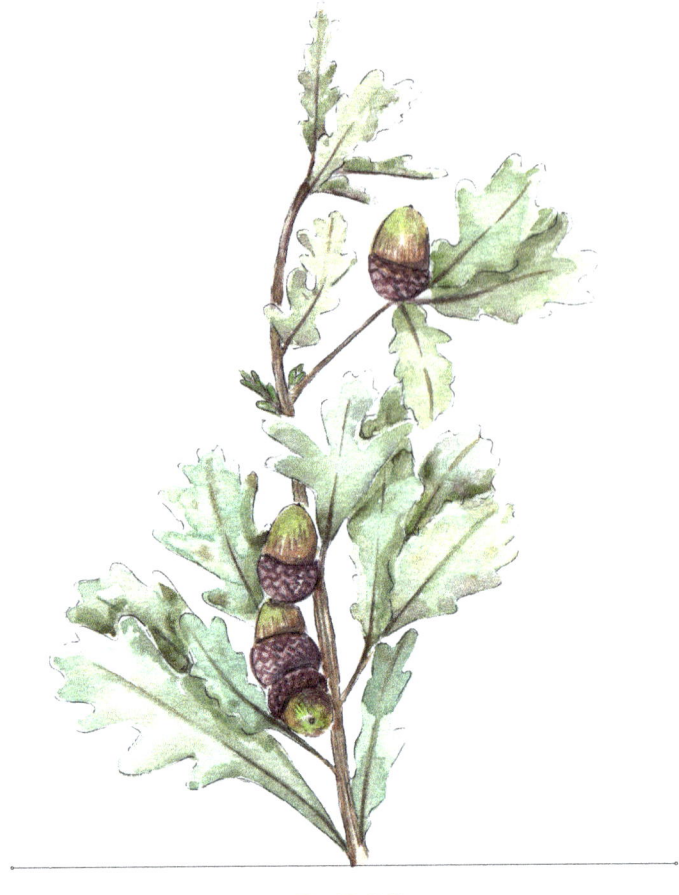

OAK

Quercus pedunculata

The Essence: The essence of Oak extract is rooted strength.

ESSENCE **ROOTED STRENGTH**	STAGE	1 - 4
	SUPER POWER	The ability to boost mental and physical energy is Oak's Super Power.
	DOSAGE	3-18 drops up to 3x daily
	AGE	From 2 years
	BEST TIME OF DAY	Anytime
	POTENTIAL PARTNERS	All acute extracts
	COMPARE WITH	Blackthorn, Black Currant
	PRECAUTIONS	If taking medication to lower blood pressure, be aware that Oak can increase blood pressure.

THE ART

Meet Oak

Oak reminds you of the strength you possess but cannot access. A gentle nudge from Oak makes that inner power more accessible, whether you need protection from viral pathogens or are recovering from a long illness, such as a cold, flu, or surgery. Think of Oak as a boost, and recognize that while it's most appreciated, it is best received in moderation. So, reach for Oak when you need its beneficial support and discontinue use once your strength is restored. It can be replaced with Blackthorn, which, through different actions, also improves states of exhaustion.

Lauren's Experience

I haven't required Oak's support often, but when I have, I am always astounded at its rapid ability to restore. It's powerful, so for my sensitive system, I have discovered that just a few days of a single dose is enough. As a practitioner, I found Oak most useful for my more mature clients who struggled to regain their physical stamina after acute episodes.

THE SCIENCE

The Actions of the Extract

Primary

Oak is helpful during the first stages of healing to support the adrenals when optimizing elimination is the goal. Its primary action is as a tonic for the adrenal glands, but it differs from Black Currant in that it acts only on the adrenal cortex. Steroids are synthesized in the adrenal cortex, so this tonic helps harmonize hormone production. Oak extract is high in antioxidants, protecting all systems from aging.

When exhaustion is a primary symptom, Oak can be added to acute protocols as needed.

Super Power

The ability to boost mental and physical energy is Oak's Super Power.

OAK NOTES:

_____

_____

_____

_____

_____

_____

_____

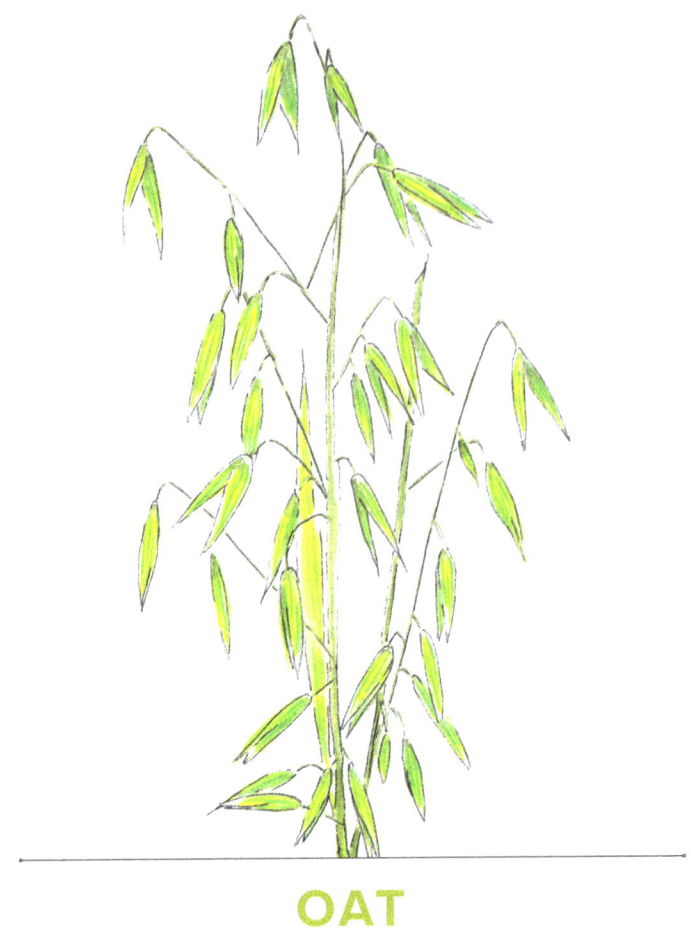

OAT

Avena sativa

The Essence: Establishing roots is the essence of Oat.

ESSENCE **ESTABLISHING ROOTS**	STAGE	2 - 4 in a microdose
	SUPER POWER	The ability to provide a stable foundation when yours is weak is Oat's Super Power.
	DOSAGE	1 drop 1x daily
	AGE	From birth
	BEST TIME OF DAY	Anytime
	POTENTIAL PARTNERS	All acute extracts
	COMPARE WITH	Dog Rose, White Willow
	PRECAUTIONS	See text

THE ART

Meet Oat

Oat is a beautiful extract to consider when you have been swept off your feet by a cold, flu, or virus that disturbs your sense of groundedness and security. Its ability to offer the re-establishment of roots can take a few days, so be patient and you will receive its reward. Its adaptogenic effects will certainly be appreciated during your weakened state.

Lauren's Experience

I love the nurturing quality Oat offers during an acute cold, flu, or virus. It reminds me to tend to myself, and its adaptogen action supports both my emotional and physical needs.

THE SCIENCE

The Actions of the Extract

Primary

Oat's primary action is to harmonize the Central and Autonomic Nervous Systems. Like the nervous system extracts Blackthorn and Silver Birch Seeds, it offers an adaptogenic effect when facing enduring or extreme physical or mental stress.

Oat offers support to the CNS in a microdose when a lack of grounding or instability is experienced during an acute viral infection.

Precautions

There is a harmonizing effect on the endocrine system, so it should not be used with medications that adjust hormone levels.

Super Power

The ability to provide a stable foundation when yours is weak is Oat's Super Power.

OAT NOTES:

_____

_____

_____

_____

_____

_____

_____

_____

SEA BUCKTHORN

Hippophae rhamnoides

The Essence: The essence of this extract is to defend the emotional and physical body.

ESSENCE **DEFEND**	STAGE	1 & 4
	SUPER POWER	The ability to shift the pH at the site of inflammation is Sea Buckthorn's Super Power.
	DOSAGE	3-18 drops up to 3x daily
	AGE	From birth
	BEST TIME OF DAY	Anytime
	POTENTIAL PARTNERS	Black Currant and all acute extracts
	COMPARE WITH	Black Poplar
	PRECAUTIONS	See text

THE ART

Meet Sea Buckthorn

Sea Buckthorn is used as soon as you notice a drop in energy, appetite, and mood to boost immune response and modify pH. It is also helpful in the convalescence stage to prevent relapses of infectious states.

Lauren's Experience

I could go on and on with my praise of Sea Buckthorn, but what stands out most to me is its ability to turn the threat of a cold, flu, or virus around IF it is used early enough following exposure. My second favorite quality of Sea Buckthorn is how it lifts my spirits, even if I must alter my schedule to slow down and tend to my symptoms. When I consider all of the extracts available, Sea Buckthorn has a place in every home and practice. I can't imagine a human or companion animal that would not benefit from its protective actions at one time or another.

THE SCIENCE

The Actions of the Extract

Primary

The primary action of Sea Buckthorn is as a tonic for the Immune System. It resolves inflammation in the early stages of colds, flus, and viruses and modifies the pH in the region of the inflammation, thus preventing pathogens from thriving.

Its tonic action for the Immune System helps resolve inflammation and modify the pH in the area of inflammation throughout the stages of an acute cold, flu, or virus.

Precautions

The high antioxidant action of this extract requires a minimum of one stool daily to prevent aggravation.

Super Power

The ability to shift the pH at the site of inflammation is Sea Buckthorn's Super Power.

SEA BUCKTHORN NOTES:

SILVER BIRCH BUDS

Betula verrucosa

The Essence: The essence of the extract made from the buds of the Silver Birch Tree is vitality.

ESSENCE VITALITY	STAGE	3 & 4
	SUPER POWER	The clearing of inflammatory conditions is Silver Birch Buds' Super Power.
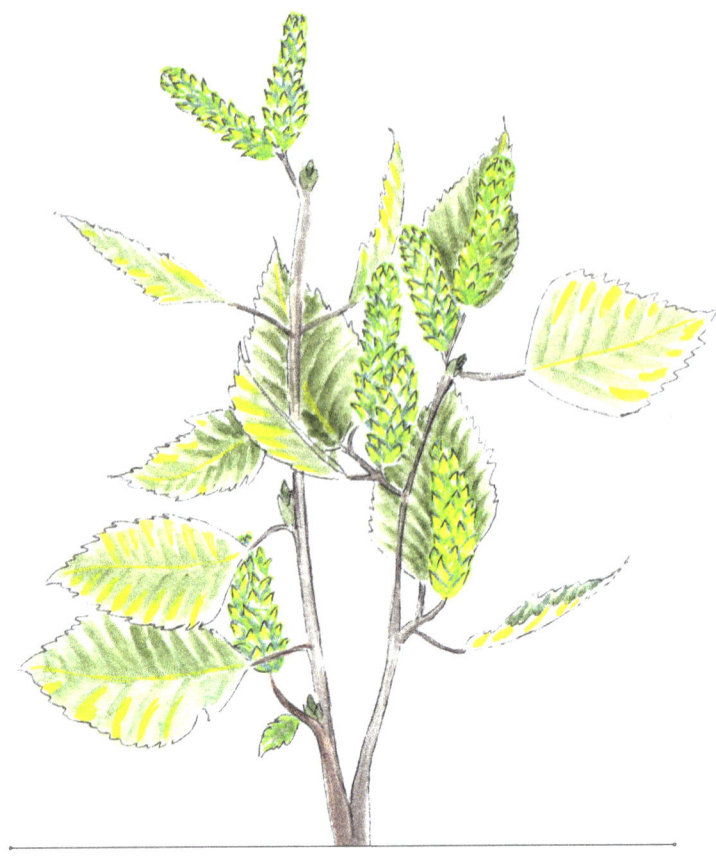	DOSAGE	3-18 drops up to 3x daily
	AGE	From birth
	BEST TIME OF DAY	Anytime
	POTENTIAL PARTNERS	Black Currant, Common Alder, Dog Rose, Lithy, Black Honeysuckle, Hazel, Hornbeam
	COMPARE WITH	Common Birch, Blackthorn
	PRECAUTIONS	No confirmed precautions at the time of publication

THE ART

Meet Silver Birch Bud

Silver Birch Bud extract supports elimination and boosts the immune response during extended cold, flu, or virus symptoms, as in Stage 3. It also plays a vital role in protocols to support Stage 4 convalescing when energy and immune response may need a boost.

Lauren's Experience

Although I don't have much personal experience with Silver Birch Buds, I often observed its restorative effects with many clients, particularly children and adults, yet in the first half of their lives.

THE SCIENCE

The Actions of the Extract

Primary

The primary action of Silver Birch Buds is as a tonic for the Immune and Respiratory Systems. It resolves acute and chronic inflammation in the mucosal lining of the respiratory system. It also inhibits the production of histamines in the lungs, digestive system, and skin, and promotes general detoxification of the body.

Its primary action as a tonic for the Immune and Respiratory systems helps resolve acute inflammation of the mucosal lining of the respiratory system.

In laboratory tests (2022), Silver Birch Bud was proven effective in creating an inhospitable environment against *Pseudomonas aeruginosa, Escherichia coli, Staphylococcus aureus* (methicillin-resistant), and *Helicobacter pylori*. Additionally, *Mycobacterium spp.* (resistant to conventional tuberculosis treatment) and *Plasmodium spp.* (resistant to classic malaria treatment).

Super Power

The clearing of inflammatory conditions is Silver Birch Buds' Super Power.

SILVER BIRCH BUD NOTES:

_____

_____

_____

_____

_____

_____

_____

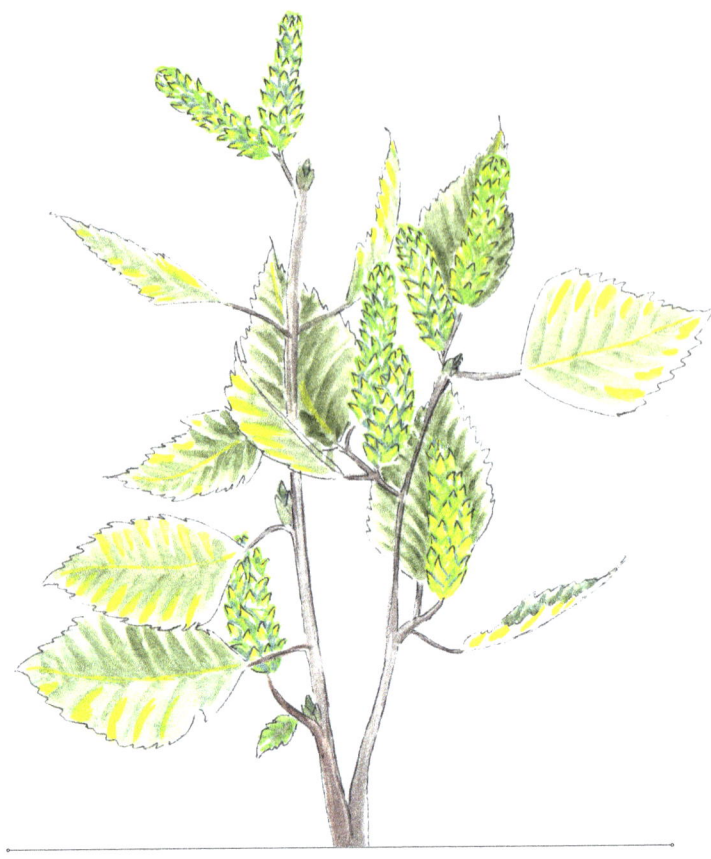

SILVER BIRCH SAP

Betula verrucosa

The Essence: The essence of Silver Birch Sap is root nourishment, with the root being the kidneys, the life force of the body.

ESSENCE NOURISHMENT	STAGE	2 - 4
	SUPER POWER	The ability of Silver Birch Sap to literally clean the skin of any residue of viral rash is its Super Power.
	DOSAGE	3-18 drops up to 3x daily
	AGE	From birth
	BEST TIME OF DAY	Anytime
	POTENTIAL PARTNERS	Black Currant
	COMPARE WITH	Common Birch, Blackthorn
	PRECAUTIONS	See text

THE ART

Meet Silver Birch Sap

Silver Birch Sap is the first extract to be considered when a rash appears during a cold, flu, or virus. Due to its tonic action, the results must be carefully monitored to avoid overworking weakened kidneys, and it should be stopped once the rash has resolved.

Lauren's Experience

I wish I had known about Silver Birch Sap decades ago, when my body often produced rashes during a viral episode. Today, however, my experience with it has been as a practitioner and mother, always amazed at how effective it can be.

THE SCIENCE

The Actions of the Extract

Primary

Silver Birch Sap has one action: tonifying the kidneys' functions. It is a mild diuretic that supports the removal of lipids, toxins, and minerals from the body.

During acute inflammatory flares of the skin, consider Silver Birch Sap as one of the first extracts for elimination support.

Precautions

It cannot be taken for indefinite periods due to the tonic effect. Signs of over-tonification include:

- An increase or return of circles under the eyes
- Lower back discomfort that was not present before beginning the extract

Special Note: Silver Birch Sap is not a true gemmotherapy extract, although it is prepared as one. It is prepared from fresh birch sap and diluted with water, alcohol, and glycerin.

Super Power

The ability of Silver Birch Sap to literally clean the skin of any residue of viral rash is its Super Power.

SILVER BIRCH SAP NOTES:

_____

_____

_____

_____

_____

SILVER LIME

Tilia tomentosa

The Essence: The essence of Silver Lime is reconnection.

ESSENCE **RECONNECTION**	STAGE	2 - 4
	SUPER POWER	The ability to restore harmonic communication between systems within your body is Silver Lime's Super Power.
	DOSAGE	1 drop once daily
	AGE	From birth
	BEST TIME OF DAY	Morning or Midday
	POTENTIAL PARTNERS	All acute extracts
	COMPARE WITH	Oats, Hops, White Willow
	PRECAUTIONS	See text

THE ART

Meet Silver Lime

While it is not the first Nervous System support extract to be taken in the case of acute symptoms, it's important to have on hand as it plays a vital role. Silver Lime offers acute, in-the-moment support for a dry, irritating cough caused by a cold, flu, or virus. It should also be considered CNS/ANS support in a microdose when disconnection is an emotional theme during an acute viral infection. True to its essence, Silver Lime is adept at reconnecting you with your inner essence and your environment.

Lauren's Experience

A long-standing cold, flu, or virus can easily lead me right into a state of disconnection that can be remedied quickly with a few days of microdosing Silver Lime.

THE SCIENCE

The Actions of the Extract

Primary

Silver Lime harmonizes the Central and Autonomic Nervous Systems by re-establishing lost connections. This work is foundational and essential in the healing process. The effects of this reconnection are calming yet not sedative.

The harmonizing effect of Silver Lime on the CNS and ANS re-establishes lost connections during an acute viral infection. **It also offers in-the-moment support for a dry, irritating cough caused by a cold, flu, or virus.**

Precautions

Although Silver Lime can be given in full doses, I recommend only microdosing for Nervous System support.

Despite its calming action, it can disrupt sleep if taken too late into the evening. Therefore, I suggest taking it only in the morning or midday.

Silver lime has been known to cause paradoxical effects, such as agitation or irritability, and overstimulation of the Nervous System. This effect is likely due to the overexcitement of receptors in the brain when intestinal dysbiosis is present. In this case, it should be combined with a microdose of Common Fig to block this response at the brain level.

Super Power

The ability to restore harmonic communication between systems within your body is Silver Lime's Super Power.

SILVER LIME NOTES:

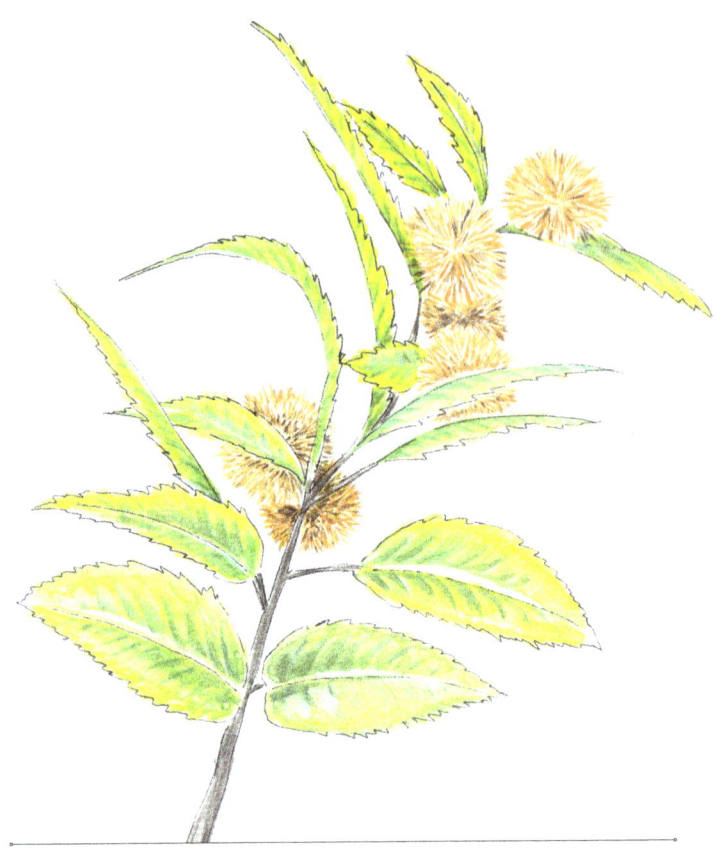

SWEET CHESTNUT

Castanea sativa

The Essence: The essence of this extract from the buds of the Sweet Chestnut tree is gentle release.

ESSENCE GENTLE RELEASE	STAGE	2 - 4
	SUPER POWER	The deep but gentle ability to move fluids is Sweet Chestnut's Super Power.
	DOSAGE	3-18 drops up to 3x daily
	AGE	From 3 years
	BEST TIME OF DAY	Anytime
	POTENTIAL PARTNERS	Horse Chestnut, Hornbeam, Common Alder, Black Currant
	COMPARE WITH	Black Poplar, Horse Chestnut
	PRECAUTIONS	No confirmed precautions at the time of publication

THE ART

Meet Sweet Chestnut

Sweet Chestnut can be considered at two distinct junctures in the healing journey and revisited as often as necessary. Think of Sweet Chestnut when acute cold, flu, and virus symptoms settle into the respiratory system, and movement of fluids is needed.

It combines well with other extracts that resolve inflammation or does well on its own, alternated with a dose of Common Alder, Black Currant, and Hornbeam or Black Honeysuckle.

Lauren's Experience

I don't need to use Sweet Chestnut often, but when I do, I am reminded of its gentle but deep effects. I consider it when I've developed a cough that is simply out of the effective range of hornbeam or lithy. I've found it to be relatively quick in its response without any aggravation despite its tonifying actions.

THE SCIENCE

The Actions of the Extract

Primary

It has a tonifying action on the Immune System that has only recently been discovered, offering protection from pathogens and antioxidant actions.

High in flavonoids, particularly quercetin and quercetin derivatives

The primary tonic action for the Immune System supports the respiratory system from onset to convalescence during an acute cold, flu, or virus.

Super Power

The deep but gentle ability to move fluids is Sweet Chestnut's Super Power.

SWEET CHESTNUT NOTES:

___
___
___
___
___
___
___
___

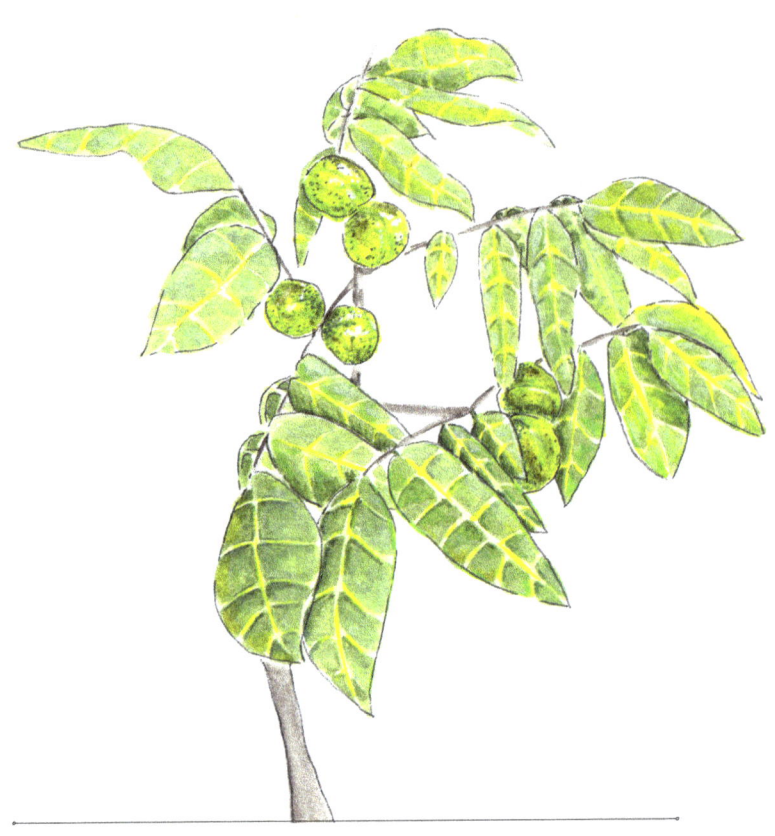

WALNUT

Juglans regia

The Essence: The essence of the extract made from the buds of the Walnut tree is shielding.

ESSENCE SHIELDING	STAGE	2 & 3
	SUPER POWER	The protection Walnut offers mucosal membranes is its Super Power.
	DOSAGE	3-18 drops up to 3x daily OR 1 drop 1x daily
	AGE	From 12 months
	BEST TIME OF DAY	Anytime
	POTENTIAL PARTNERS	Best alone
	COMPARE WITH	Fig
	PRECAUTIONS	See text

THE ART

Meet Walnut

Always consider Walnut when there is inflammation of the digestive tract during a cold, flu, or virus, or as an adjunct support for the mucosal lining of the digestive tract when taking antibiotics. It can also be used topically for inflamed skin wounds and as protection against radiation during flights, dental X-rays, and radiation therapy.

Lauren's Experience

When it comes to cold, flu, and virus symptoms, Walnut plays a role when the inflammation is in the digestive tract. In that case, as is advised with all uses of Walnut, I take it separately from other extracts. As mentioned in this description, I use Walnut a great deal as a first aid treatment for cuts, abrasions, and burns. Its ability to heal skin along with its antimicrobial properties makes it one of my favorite travel extracts.

THE SCIENCE

The Actions of the Extract

Primary

Walnut has two primary actions. The first action is as a Tonic resolving infectious states that occur on a mucosal level. This action applies to the digestive system, the urinary system, the vagina, and all skin surfaces.

Secondary

Walnut also acts as a Harmonizer for the CNS.

The tonic action of Walnut helps resolve infectious states that occur on a mucosal level or topically for skin inflammation, and for the CNS when withdrawing from society seems most comfortable.

Precautions

When using it in a protocol with other extracts, take the Walnut dose separately at a different time of day.

Walnut Gemmo extract is made from the tree's leaf buds and is safe for those who have an allergy to the nut itself.

Super Power

The protection Walnut offers mucosal membranes is its Super Power.

WALNUT NOTES:

_____

_____

_____

_____

_____

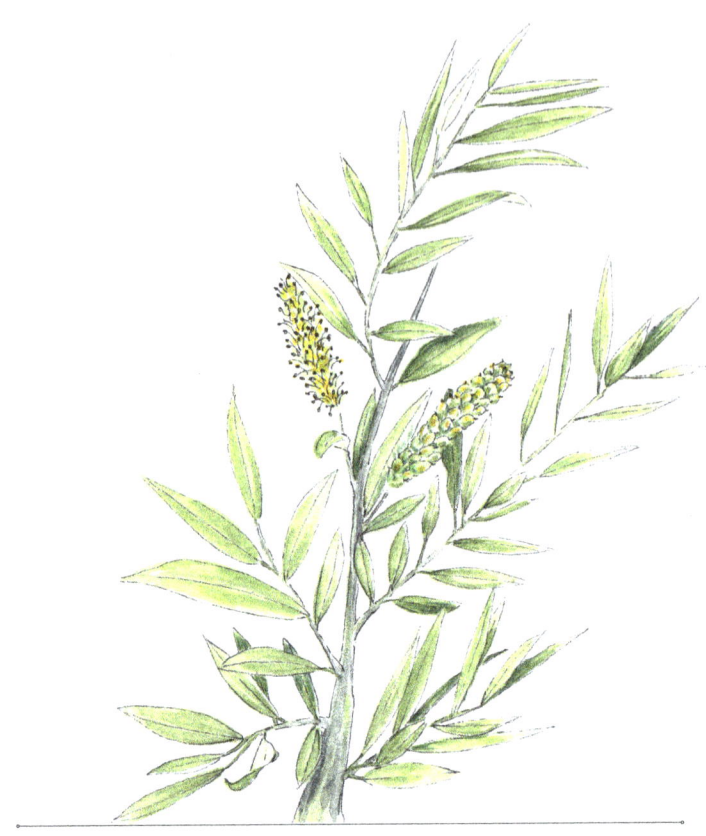

WHITE WILLOW

Salix alba

The Essence: The essence of this extract from the buds of the White Willow is gathering.

ESSENCE GATHERING	STAGE	2 - 4 only as CNS support
	SUPER POWER	The ability to restore ease to a harried state is White Willow's Super Power.
	DOSAGE	1 drop 1x daily
	AGE	From 6 years
	BEST TIME OF DAY	Anytime
	POTENTIAL PARTNERS	All acute extracts
	COMPARE WITH	Dog Rose, Oat
	PRECAUTIONS	Not to be used by individuals who are allergic to aspirin

THE ART

Meet White Willow

Think of White Willow each morning in a microdose to support you through a harried state to one of ease anytime during stages 2-4. Perhaps you are experiencing overwhelm from all that you can not attend to during this illness, or you are still trying to care for others while attempting to recover yourself. If you find this state prevents you from easing into sleep, consider taking it once each evening instead of the morning.

Lauren's Experience

I wish I could share a glowing review of White Willow but to date my only experience is not so pleasant. I have an allergic reaction to salicin compound found in willow and even one drop of White Willow causes painful inflammation — just the opposite of its desired effect. I believe it is important to have these reactions from time to time so that I can confidently share that it should be avoided by all with an aspirin allergy.

THE SCIENCE

The Actions of the Extract

Primary

The primary action of Salix alba is as a Harmonizer for the Central and Autonomic Nervous Systems. It has a harmonizing action on the neurotransmitter acetylcholine and is mildly sedating.

The harmonizing action on the CNS makes White Willow an excellent choice for feelings of overwhelm and a sense that you cannot protect yourself during an acute viral infection.

Super Power

The ability to restore ease to a harried state is White Willow's Super Power.

WHITE WILLOW NOTES:

_____

_____

_____

_____

_____

_____

_____

SUMMARY OF NOTED PRECAUTIONS FOR ACUTE PROTOCOLS

EXTRACT	KNOWN PRECAUTIONS
BLACK HONEYSUCKLE	Avoid if the liver is congested.
BLACK POPLAR	Avoid if taking anti-coagulants, anti-platelets, or daily aspirin.
BLACKTHORN	Begin with a microdose.
COMMON ALDER	Avoid during breastfeeding and pregnancy; use only in combination with other extracts
FIELD MAPLE	As with all extracts for the liver, begin with a small dose and watch for aggravations such as irritability or hives.
HOPS	Avoid during breastfeeding and pregnancy; Short-term use only; Estrogenic effect; Avoid when using hormone-balancing medications.
HORNBEAM	Avoid if taking anti-coagulants, anti-platelets, daily aspirin. Should not be taken for more than 4 to 6 weeks.
HORSE CHESTNUT	Avoid if taking anti-coagulants, anti-platelets, daily aspirin
LINGONBERRY	Not recommended for individuals with suspicion of or diagnosed with estrogen-dependent cancers.
LITHY	It can slow stool elimination, so combine it with a well-matched elimination extract when taking it daily.
MAGNOLIA	Avoid during breastfeeding and pregnancy. Use only in combination with other extracts.
OAK	Could raise blood pressure.
OAT	Avoid when using hormone-balancing medications.
SEA BUCKTHORN	The high antioxidant action of this extract requires a minimum of one stool daily to prevent aggravation.
SILVER BIRCH SAP	Cannot be taken for indefinite periods due to the tonic effect. Signs of over-tonification include: An increase or return of circles under the eyes and/or lower back discomfort that was not present before beginning the extract
SILVER LIME	Although Silver Lime can be given in full doses, I recommend only microdosing for Nervous System support. Despite its calming action, it can disrupt sleep if taken too late into the evening. Therefore, I suggest taking it only in the morning or midday. Has been known to cause paradoxical effects, such as agitation or irritability, and over-stimulation of the Nervous System. This effect is likely due to the overexcitement of receptors in the brain when intestinal dysbiosis is present. In this case, it should be combined with a microdose of Common Fig to block this response at the brain level.
WALNUT	When using it in a protocol with other extracts, take the Walnut dose separately at a different time of day. The extract is made from the tree's leaf buds and is safe for those who have an allergy to the nut itself.
WHITE WILLOW	Not to be used by individuals who are allergic to aspirin.

POSSIBLE AGGRAVATIONS

Possible Emotional Aggravations from Nervous System Extracts

IRRITABILITY	Occurs when a tonic action aggravates the liver. Choose a different Central Nervous System (CNS) extract to microdose. Try this extract again in 1 to 2 weeks after using other extracts and observe your reaction.
INCREASED ANXIETY	Occurs when there is a paradoxical effect, often due to disharmony within the digestive system. Add an extract to support the digestive system/eliminationand try again after 5-7 days.
SADNESS	Can occur when an extract for the nervous system uncovers a layer that has been suppressed. Observe if the symptoms are increasing or decreasing. If it increases, choose a different CNS extract to microdose. Try this extract again 1-2 weeks after using other extracts and observe your reaction.
DISTURBING DREAMS	It can occur when a particular emotion or part of yourself has recently been suppressed. This part needs your attention; if you don't tend to it during the day, it will arrive through your subconscious at night. You can choose another CNS extract for now; however, I suggest you consider what is being asked of you when you have gained some resilience and then try the extract again.

Possible Physical Reactions from all extracts

SKIN INFLAMMATION—HIVES OR RASH	This is most likely associated with taking too much of an extract that affects the liver. Skip taking it until the inflammation improves. Then, choose a different extract or reduce the amount dosed by half. If it is still an issue, try taking it every other day.
DIGESTIVE DISTURBANCES	This is most likely associated with taking too much of an extract that has a tonic action on a part of the digestive system. Skip taking it one day and reduce the amount dosed by half.
LOWER BACK DISCOMFORT	This is most likely associated with taking too much of an extract that has a tonic action on the kidneys. Skip taking it one day and reduce the amount dosed by half.
PAIN IN JOINTS	This is most likely associated with taking too much of an extract that has a tonic action on the kidneys. Skip taking it one day and reduce the amount dosed by half.
DISTURBED SLEEP	This is most likely associated with an extract that has a tonic action that has been taken to late in the day or the dose is too high. Usually, this occurs with extracts that support digestion/elimination. Skip taking it one day and try again late morning instead of midday or afternoon, or reduce the amount dosed by half.

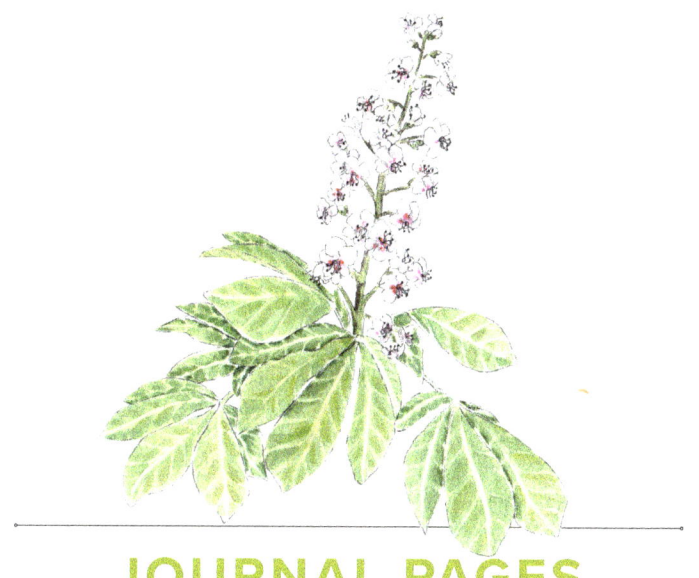

JOURNAL PAGES

Taking the time to record and reflect on your personal experiences will not only help you better understand the acute care stages, but it will also strengthen your relationship with each Gemmo Extract used.

NAME	DATE

SYMPTOM FIRST NOTICED:

OBSERVATIONS OF THE FOLLOWING:

MOOD	ENERGY LEVEL	APPETITE

OTHER SYMPTOMS, AND THE DATES THEY OCCUR:

EYES, EARS, NOSE	FEVER, BODY ACHES	RASH
THROAT, COUGH	NAUSEA, VOMITING, LOOSE STOOLS	OTHER

THE PROTOCOL:

STAGE ONE	STAGE TWO	STAGE THREE	STAGE FOUR

Taking the time to record and reflect on your personal experiences will not only help you better understand the acute care stages, but it will also strengthen your relationship with each Gemmo Extract used.

NAME

DATE

SYMPTOM FIRST NOTICED

OBSERVATIONS OF THE FOLLOWING:

MOOD

ENERGY LEVEL

APPETITE

OTHER SYMPTOMS, AND THE DATES THEY OCCUR:

EYES, EARS, NOSE

FEVER, BODY ACHES

RASH

THROAT, COUGH

NAUSEA, VOMITING, LOOSE STOOLS

OTHER

THE PROTOCOL:

STAGE ONE

STAGE TWO

STAGE THREE

STAGE FOUR

Taking the time to record and reflect on your personal experiences will not only help you better understand the acute care stages, but it will also strengthen your relationship with each Gemmo Extract used.

NAME

DATE

SYMPTOM FIRST NOTICED

OBSERVATIONS OF THE FOLLOWING:

MOOD

ENERGY LEVEL

APPETITE

OTHER SYMPTOMS, AND THE DATES THEY OCCUR:

EYES, EARS, NOSE

FEVER, BODY ACHES

RASH

THROAT, COUGH

NAUSEA, VOMITING, LOOSE STOOLS

OTHER

THE PROTOCOL:

STAGE ONE

STAGE TWO

STAGE THREE

STAGE FOUR

Taking the time to record and reflect on your personal experiences will not only help you better understand the acute care stages, but it will also strengthen your relationship with each Gemmo Extract used.

NAME

DATE

SYMPTOM FIRST NOTICED

OBSERVATIONS OF THE FOLLOWING:

MOOD

ENERGY LEVEL

APPETITE

OTHER SYMPTOMS, AND THE DATES THEY OCCUR:

EYES, EARS, NOSE

FEVER, BODY ACHES

RASH

THROAT, COUGH

NAUSEA, VOMITING, LOOSE STOOLS

OTHER

THE PROTOCOL:

STAGE ONE

STAGE TWO

STAGE THREE

STAGE FOUR

Taking the time to record and reflect on your personal experiences will not only help you better understand the acute care stages, but it will also strengthen your relationship with each Gemmo Extract used.

NAME	DATE

SYMPTOM FIRST NOTICED

OBSERVATIONS OF THE FOLLOWING:

MOOD	ENERGY LEVEL	APPETITE

OTHER SYMPTOMS, AND THE DATES THEY OCCUR:

EYES, EARS, NOSE	FEVER, BODY ACHES	RASH
THROAT, COUGH	NAUSEA, VOMITING, LOOSE STOOLS	OTHER

THE PROTOCOL:

STAGE ONE	STAGE TWO	STAGE THREE	STAGE FOUR

Taking the time to record and reflect on your personal experiences will not only help you better understand the acute care stages, but it will also strengthen your relationship with each Gemmo Extract used.

NAME

DATE

SYMPTOM FIRST NOTICED

OBSERVATIONS OF THE FOLLOWING:

MOOD

ENERGY LEVEL

APPETITE

OTHER SYMPTOMS, AND THE DATES THEY OCCUR:

EYES, EARS, NOSE

FEVER, BODY ACHES

RASH

THROAT, COUGH

NAUSEA, VOMITING LOOSE STOOLS

OTHER

THE PROTOCOL:

STAGE ONE

STAGE TWO

STAGE THREE

STAGE FOUR

www.ingramcontent.com/pod-product-compliance
Lightning Source LLC
Chambersburg PA
CBHW080550030426
42337CB00024B/4829